Akak'stiman

Akak'stiman

A Blackfoot Framework for Decision-Making and Mediation Processes

Reg Crowshoe and Sybille Manneschmidt

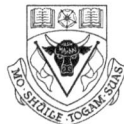

UNIVERSITY OF
CALGARY
PRESS

University of Calgary Press
2500 University Drive NW
Calgary, Alberta
Canada T2N 1N4
www.uofcpress.com

National Library of Canada Cataloguing in Publication Data

Crowshoe, Reg.
Akak'stiman

Includes bibliographical references.
ISBN 1-55238-044-0
1. Piegan Indians—Medical care. 2. Siksika Indians—Medical care. 3. Medical care—Alberta. 4. Traditional medicine—Alberta. 5. Piegan Indians—Rites and ceremonies. 6. Siksika Indians—Rites and ceremonies. 7. Piegan Indians—Medicine. 8. Siksika Indians—Medicine. I. Manneschmidt, Sybille, 1952- II. Title.

E99.P58C76 2002   362.1'089'97307123   C2002-910099-2

Canada

We acknowledge the financial support of the Government of Canada through the Book Publishing Industry Development Program (BPIDP) for our publishing activities.

The Canada Council for the Arts
Le Conseil des Arts du Canada

Front cover photo: NA 118-16, courtesy of Glenbow Archives, Calgary
All royalties received through this publication will be transferred to the Joe and Josephine Crowshoe Foundation, Calgary.

Page, cover design, and typesetting by Kristina Schuring.

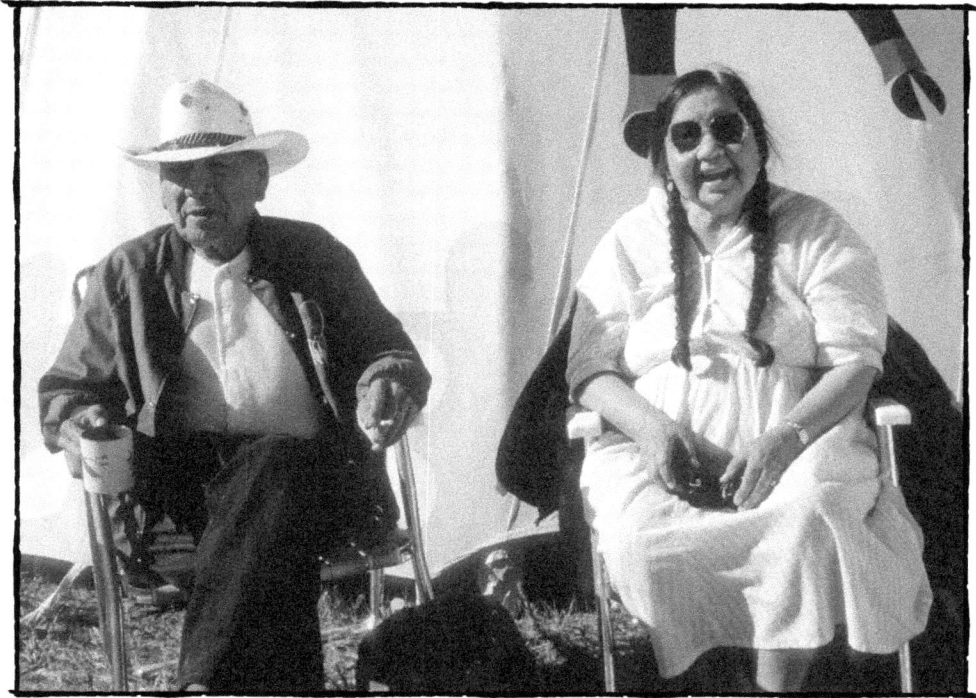

This text is dedicated to our teachers, Joe and Josephine Crowshoe.

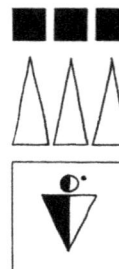

Introduction to the Second Edition

Akak'stiman is a Blackfoot term meaning "law-making." It relates to the one annual event in the seasonal cycle of Blackfoot culture when all people came together to celebrate the Sun Dance ceremony and witness the making and enforcement of their laws. Today, the Sun Dance is still in most Blackfoot nations an integral part of spiritual celebrations. But unlike in the past, this event is not anymore the coming together of all clans and has lost its social function of representing unity and strength of the various Blackfoot-speaking groups.

Since the beginning of the research on this book in 1992 (and its first publication in 1997), the Blackfoot Circle Structure model has been implemented in various settings. The new edition embraces these newer developments.

Consequently, the following text varies in certain aspects from the original version. The first edition focused on the health-related history of the Peigan people, present-day health issues, and a health-management model that is built on the Blackfoot Circle Structure's principles.

This edition will extend its focus to offer other potential applications of this model in decision-making and mediation processes. Accordingly, certain changes have been made to the original text, and they are primarily to be found in Chapter 9. We hope that these additions will offer the reader a better understanding of the application of this management model and that we are able to demonstrate its value in interpreting Western practices to Native peoples whose collective past evolved around circular structures.

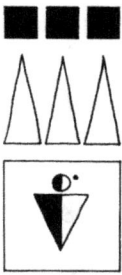

Summary

Health is one of many cultural constructions in human society. This document deals with the present-day health structures of a group of Native peoples in Canada, the residents of the Peigan Reserve in southern Alberta. The presented research will show that there are two health systems in place: one based on traditional Blackfoot culture and a second that has developed since the establishment of Indian reserves—in this case since about the turn of the century.

The historical Blackfoot health system emphasizes the survival of the individual within the group and is grounded in traditional Blackfoot ceremonial processes that have been practised over hundreds of years. The other, newer, medical model is based on Western theories of illness and curing. Health services are provided by both models. However, the latter method is the only one endorsed by the government bureaucracies. Peigan traditional health services, by contrast, are a private choice.

This document describes the importance of traditional Blackfoot health services and their foundation in age-old ceremonies. The following chapters give some background information on these ceremonies, which have shaped both the past and present traditional health services. It is the researchers' aim to show that these ceremonies provide a specific framework for decision-making that can be used as a model for present-day health service delivery. The study concludes that this model could be successfully used as a tool for discussion forums for both Western and traditional Blackfoot health services systems, with the potential to provide improved services for the Peigan community.

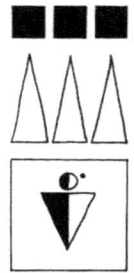

Acknowledgments

This text is the result of ongoing research related to the Keep Our Circle Strong Project, Peigan Reserve, Alberta.

In many ways, this text is based on a truly collaborative process between two individuals: Reg Crowshoe, whose years of study have resulted in the development of the Blackfoot Circle Structure model and whose contributions were the basis for this report, and Sybille Manneschmidt, who contributed her knowledge and experience as a health professional and wrote the majority of the text. However, others need to be thanked for their assistance. Heather Crowshoe submitted material for Chapter 6, Helen Little Moustache compiled some of the data for the Bibliography, and Henrietta Yellow Horn wrote Appendix B. Henrietta Yellow Horn was also the research assistant for the duration of the project, and in many

ways was the pillar of this project. Without her ongoing commitment and assistance, this project could not have been completed within its narrow timeline.

Last but not least, we thank the following organizations and agencies for their contributions: Peigan Health Administration, Treaty 7 Tribal Council, Alberta Health Aboriginal Health Strategy, Regional Centre for Health Promotion and Community Studies (RCHPCS), the University of Lethbridge, and the Department of Community Development, Government of Alberta, for their financial support; and the Old Man River Cultural Centre former and present staff, the Glenbow Museum and Archives, the Provincial Museum of Alberta, the Provincial Archives of Alberta, and the Canadian Heritage Division for their support in kind.

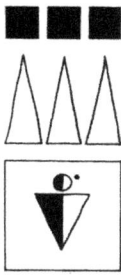

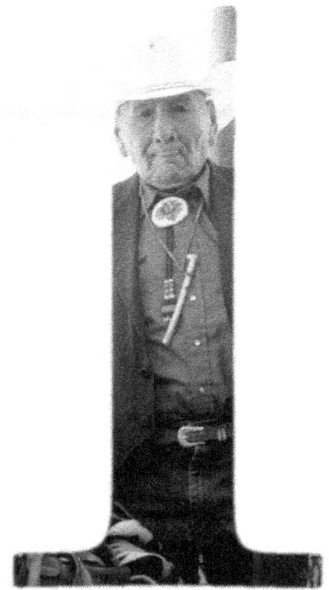

Introduction

Elders of the Peigan Nation came together in 1991 to discuss a serious situation involving the young people of their community. That year, there were several suicides committed by youths, and, of five deaths in six months, four were young people. The elders recognized that the deaths were a direct result of confusion about cultural identity and the young people's inability to cope with the realities of their community. Cultural confusion combined with alcohol and drug abuse had made them unable to deal with their lives.

Elders were concerned that the sacred traditional Blackfoot teachings were being misconstrued by some Peigan youth. They had learned ideas from people and places outside of Peigan culture that had neither the proper understanding nor certification to speak on these matters. These teachings were confusing the youth, who, once they returned to the reserve and tried to practice or implement these "unauthorized"[1] teachings, were faced with rejection and obstacles that led to frustration, anger, depression, and, too often, suicide.

The term "cultural confusion" refers to how these young people perceived concepts of personal power and traditional medicine, which in the elders' eyes were misunderstood. As the following chapters will point out, traditional Blackfoot culture understands "power" as being in the Creator only and in some of Creation's representations. "Power" and "medicine,"[2] therefore, are not located in or owned by a person. Power/medicine can be accessed with the help of a skilfully trained individual who has gone through cultural training and accreditation.

The 1991 discussions by the elders led to the Keep Our Circle Strong Project, which started with the intention of bringing traditional teachings to the fore, and specifically to the notice of Peigan youth. Since that time, the Project has, based on historical and ethnographic research, developed the Blackfoot Circle Structure Process. This model is used as a venue "to translate" traditional Blackfoot concepts and apply these to the present-day life of Peigan people. Reg Crowshoe has been involved since the beginning in this process of translation and implementation, and several applications have been put into practice in the past years. These are the Peigan Sentencing Circle program and educational and tourism programs.

However, this is the first time that the Blackfoot Circle Structure model is presented in text form. In this case, it has been applied to three specific areas: health administration and services mediation processes in child protection, and corporate processes of decision-making.

The need to develop a health-related application of the Blackfoot Circle Structure model derived from the researchers' realization that: (a) individual and collective health behaviours are related to traditional Blackfoot cultural aspects, and (b) the present-day political situation (with the question of self-government on the table and the push for takeover of health services by all

First Nations) requires a definition of how the Peigan community's traditional cultural roots have affected and can be part of health services.[3]

The other two areas of application developed out of the need of existing agencies and businesses to develop a working relationship with Blackfoot and other First Nations groups.

This book therefore has the following objectives:

- To show that traditional Peigan/Blackfoot structures have as much depth of knowledge and historical relevance as any Western structural systems, especially in the area of health delivery
- To demonstrate that this model is based on a paradigm that differs from Western systems by allowing all participants to take part equally in the process
- To propose an entry point for practical application

The following report has no intention of persuading anyone to change his or her personal belief systems. It offers an option for the Peigan community to use traditional structures in a translated form for present-day application for the benefit of their community.

Also, it does not reveal sacred information known only to initiated ceremonialists. Rather, it employs abstract concepts based on ceremonial materials and rituals that we will describe. They are essential to an understanding of the Circle Structure model and some of the traditional Peigan cultural values. (For example, important ceremonial and social status is linked with an individual's obligations and responsibilities to the community).

Background Information

The Peigan Nation comprises about 2,700 members, with the majority of the population living on a reserve in southern Alberta, Canada. The Peigan belong to the Blackfoot Confederacy, which consists of four different member nations and is part of the Treaty 7 group, which signed this agreement with representatives of Queen Victoria in 1877. The four Blackfoot nations are the Blood (Kainai), North Peigan (Aputosi Piikani), and Blackfoot (Siksika), all located in Alberta, Canada; and the South Peigan (Amaskapi Piikani, Blackfeet, or Peigan) in Montana, U.S.A. In this text, *North Peigan (Aputosi Piikani)* will refer to the group of people this book is primarily concerned with, and *Blackfeet (Amaskapi Piikani)* to the nation in the United States. When both groups are discussed, they will be referred to as *Peigan. Northern Blackfoot* is the term used for the Siksika and *Blood* for the Kainai, and when all four are mentioned the name *Blackfoot* will be used.

All authors who studied the Confederacy peoples' languages and linguistic aspects of their culture agree that all four are dialect variations of one major language, which is of Algonquian origin (Curtis 1970, de Josslin de Jong 1914, Frantz and Russell 1989, Grinnell 1892, Morgan 1964, Tims 1889, Uhlenbeck 1911, Wissler 1911). Because of the dialectic differences among the various tribal groups and among individuals, the writers' phonetic biases, based on their cultural backgrounds (for example, Dutch), and the difficulties of consistently transcribing an oral language using a foreign (English-language) alphabet, some of the words used in this text will not be found to exist in or be consistent with published Blackfoot texts. However, an effort has been made to keep the spelling of Blackfoot language terms consistent throughout this book.

Methodology

The focus of this study is the period between 1730 and 1930, which includes the so-called horse days as well as the early reservation period. Information on Blackfoot people began to be recorded around 1730, but more detailed data emerged at the end of the nineteenth century. Interviews with present-day elders who were raised by their grandparents also shed light on the period from around 1840 to the present.

Although this book focuses on the North Peigan people, material from other Blackfoot peoples has been used to supplement the available

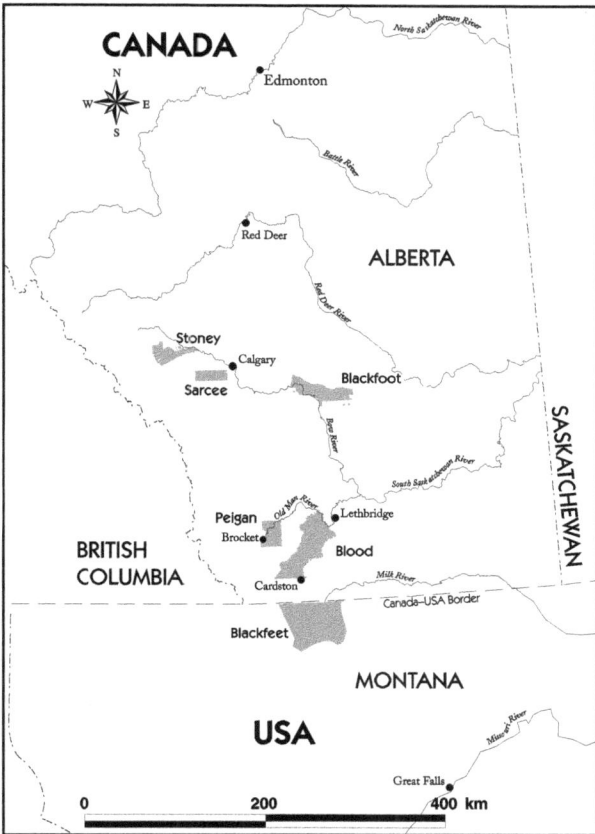

Blackfoot confederacy and Treaty 7 reservations.

people, biases that influence what kind of things are told, how they are told, what is omitted, and how things are categorized.[4] All this shapes how and in what context certain information is presented. Although sometimes events are reported in a specific light to intentionally produce a certain picture,[5] most of the time, human memory is unconsciously shaped.[6] In the history of Native peoples, this can be seen by the white men,[7] who were first to meet the Blackfoot people, reported on the role of women, the position of leaders, and religious activities, showing their personal preferences and convictions.[8]

Similarly, both researchers' selective viewpoints have shaped this report. One is a member of the Peigan Nation and long-standing ceremonialist who has been educated since his childhood in the traditional ways of his people. The other is an immigrant and academic who has worked with the North Peigan people for more than twelve years and has had the privilege of learning about many aspects of Peigan culture. This research draws on their collective experience.

This book is neither exhaustive nor complete in its historical and sociological aspects. But these aspects of Blackfoot culture need to be shown in order to understand that health and medicine are cultural constructs like any other aspect of human life.

Thus, this book has a very specific goal: an attempt to offer a structural approach for present-day North Peigan administration models deriving from traditional Blackfoot cultural practices.

data on the North Peigan. This material primarily describes the Blackfeet, as they were once part of the same tribe as the various North Peigan bands. Additionally, information from the Blood as well as the Northern Blackfoot was used when available and appropriate. For example, Wissler, who worked with the Blackfeet around the turn of the century when they were completely settled on their reservations, was one of the most important sources in developing a systematic picture of Peigan culture. Around 1950, enough oldtimers were still alive to tell stories and share their experiences from the pre-reservation and horse days. Additionally, Clark Wissler had a long-time associate and field assistant, David Charles Duvall, who was living on the Blackfeet reserve, had a Peigan mother, and spoke the language fluently.

However, these sources have specific biases, no matter if they come from Native or non-Native

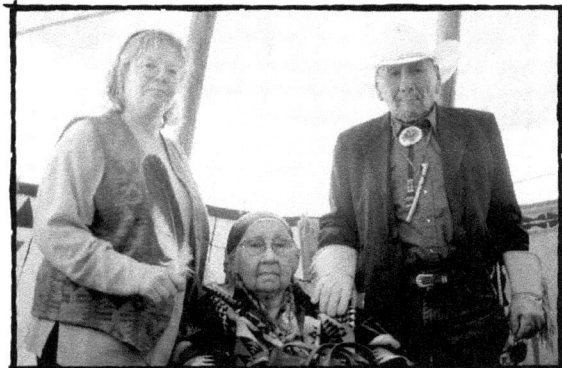

Co-author Sybille with her adoptive parents, Joe and Josephine Crowshoe on the Peigan Reserve.

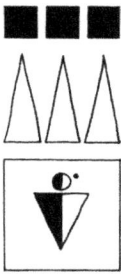

History of the Peigan People

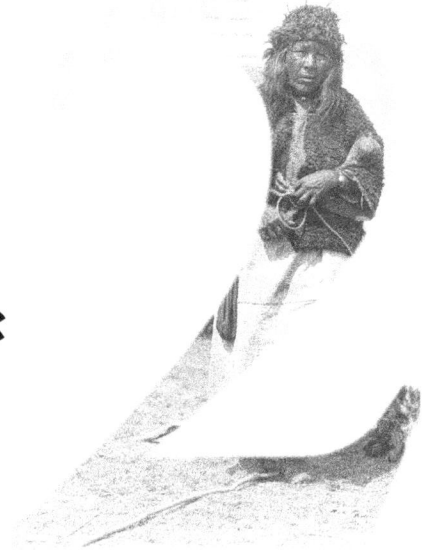

This chapter deals with the interpretation of Peigan history from a Peigan/Blackfoot as well as a Canadian/European perspective. Historical information plays an important part in shedding light on specific health issues and how Native and non-Native health systems were implemented to serve the Peigan population.

Interpretations presented in this chapter will derive from written reports by travellers (e.g., Maximilian zu Wied), explorers (e.g., Palliser), traders and Hudson Bay or North West Company employees (e.g., Fidler), members of the NWMP[1] (e.g., Nevitt), and missionaries and government officials (e.g., Doucet). These accounts stretch over a period from 1690 to 1930, covering nearly two hundred and fifty years. Although the information is sketchy in places and obviously biased by the viewpoint of the writer, it uncovers valuable data.

Another set of information comes from four sources: (1) Blackfoot wintercounts, (2) interviews and observations reported by ethnographers who started visiting the Peigan/Blackfeet around the turn of the century and had knowledgeable Blackfoot informants,[2] (3) interviews conducted in the last thirty-five years by non-professional Peigan with their elders,[3] and (4) writings by Blackfoot people themselves.[4]

A wintercount was a traditional Blackfoot documentation of specific events happening over several years, told at specific occasions or painted in symbols on a hide, something like a calendar. These symbols reflected either personal, band, or tribal events and were sometimes handed on over several years by record keepers, Blackfoot officials who also held the position of camp crier, or announcer of certain events. For this study, these accounts present information on the occurrence and patterns of disease and aspects of health that are defined as exceptional events, for example, homicides and suicides. Raczka (1979) published a wintercount (1764 to 1924) of the North Peigan tribe, as told by Bull Plume to William Haynes, an Anglican missionary who lived among the Blackfoot people for fifty-six years. Another wintercount (1810 to 1889) published by Middleton (1953) is from Father of Many Children or Bad Head, a noted band chief from the Blood. This account was originally collected by Emile Legal, an Oblate missionary, and R.N. Wilson, a former NWMP officer and later Indian agent, and was also published at a later time by Dempsey (1965). McClintock (1935) quotes from a wintercount (1836 to 1877), but it is unclear where and when he collected this information. There is knowledge about four other more recent wintercounts recorded by Native writers in reservation times, the most extensive being the wintercount of Running Rabbit (1830 to 1937), a North Blackfoot.

Usually, historians of Plains Indians categorize time by various events that affected the life of these peoples. For the Peigan/Blackfoot, the following categories will be employed: pre-historic times, the dog days, the horse days,[5] early reservation/treaty period, and early twentieth century. It is the treaty period and the subsequent settlement on the reserves by the turn of the century that are mainly reflected by collected information on Canadian government health service delivery through non-Native sources and the Indian agent bureaucracy. But the period before these interventions is also of interest to this book. As the following chapters will point out, it is the pre-reservation period from which data are still available that affected certain concepts and social structures in Peigan culture. This time exerted influence over the understanding of traditional health concepts and the development of traditional health service delivery, underscoring the importance at background information on the Peigan people's history.

Prehistoric Times

Creation stories[6] of the ancestors of present-day Blackfoot describe those ancestors as living in an area located between the Rocky Mountains in the west, the present-day province of Saskatchewan to the east, the Northern Saskatchewan River in the north, and the Upper Missouri in the United States in the south.

Some archaeologists believe that they came as prehistoric hunters across the Bering Strait more than twelve thousand years ago. Linguists connect the tribes Peigan, Blood, and Northern Blackfoot with the Algonquian language, and this is the reason why historians claim that the Blackfoot migrated from the woodland regions of Saskatchewan to the prairies.

The Peigan separated at an unknown time into North and South Peigan (Blackfeet), with the South Peigan living in present-day Montana and the North Peigan in Canada. This separation was already established before 1855, when James Doty (Dempsey 1964) mentioned a visit with several camps of North Peigan, but the tribal division was finally enforced after the Lame Bull Treaty was signed by the Blackfeet with the United States government.

Long before Alexander Henry's time in the Northwest, a part of the Ahpaitupi (Blood People) gens of the Pikuni separated from the tribe, and lived for the greater part of the time close up to the foot of the Rockies, between the St. Mary's river and the South Branch of the Saskatchewan. Henry named them the 'Cold Band'; doubtless because their chief at that time was named Ustoyimstan (Cold Maker). Eventually they became the Aputositupi (North People), or, more properly, Aputosi Pikuni (North Peigan), North Peigans of the Canadian Government. (Schultz 1930, p. 26)

When the Blackfoot people first met with white traders, they had already fully adapted to the plains culture,[7] living primarily on the buffalo.

Dog Days

This is the period before Blackfoot people acquired horses and guns using dogs with travois for transport. Buffalo were the economic base of survival for the ancestors of the present-day North Peigan people, providing food and shelter, essential raw materials for tools, storage containers, and clothes, and additional sources for trading. Because buffalo had specific seasonal patterns of movement as well as specific individual behaviours in the herd, various Indian peoples developed certain systemic approaches to hunting the buffalo. One was the famous drives of herds of buffalo over cliffs, primarily during the fall and occasionally during the spring.[8] the fact that the buffalo was the central animal to the Blackfoot is reflected in the people's mythologies and religious ceremonies as well as in their individual and group social structures. For example, the use of buffalo stones[9] in religious ceremonies and medicine bundles (Wissler 1912) and the central and ancient ritual of the Okan (Sun Dance) are only some of the evidence showing how important the buffalo were to the survival of the people.[10] The roles of leaders, gender-specific roles for men and women, and the development of the most important social structures can be clearly connected to the buffalo. Chiefs were respected for

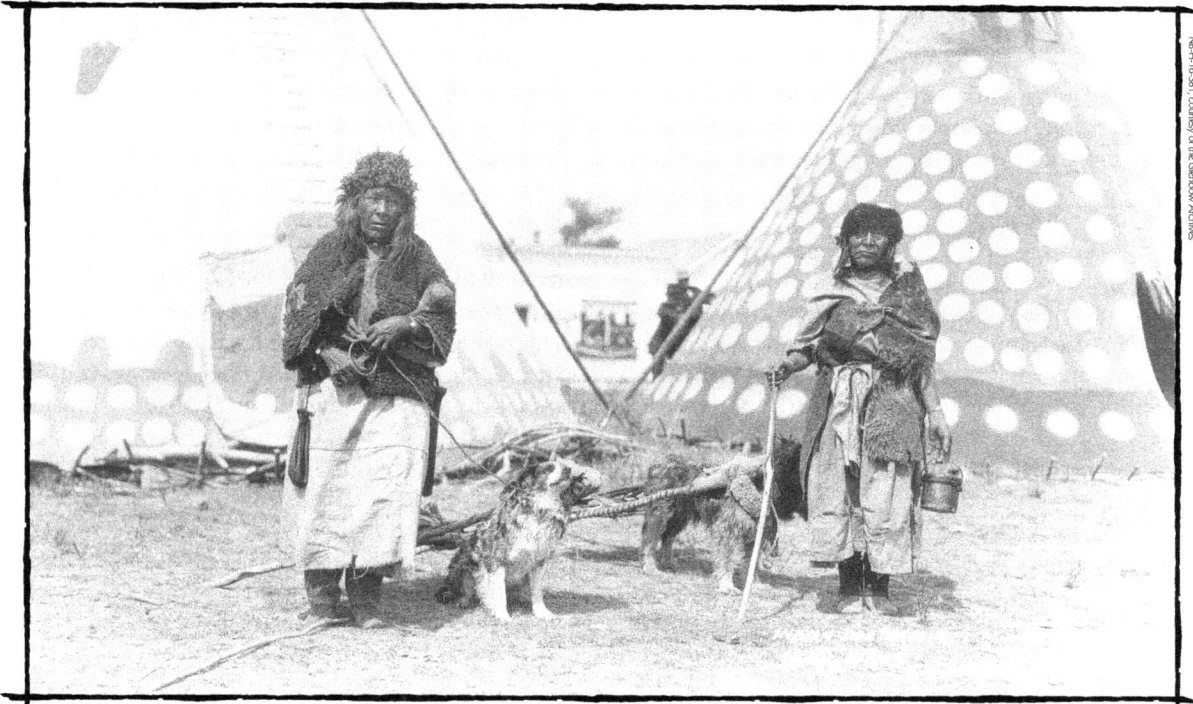

NB-H-16-381, courtesy of the Glenbow Archives

Blood women with dog travois in front of tipis, at the Calgary Exhibition and Stampede, Calgary, Alberta.

their knowledge of the migration patterns of buffalo, animal behaviour, and the lay of the land, and for their skills in instructing and supervising buffalo drives and pounds. This leads to the assumption that the old chiefs were probably Beaver bundle owners. Soldiers like the Brave Dogs had to ensure discipline (of all people involved) during the buffalo hunt. (See Chapter 3 on Social Structures.) A woman who was an efficient worker was highly respected in her culture because women did most of the processing of meat, hides, and robes. They also made the staple food, pemmican, which ensured that people could travel for a long time without depending on hunting or gathering for fresh supplies and was the only physical insurance of survival during periods of food shortage. Additionally, pemmican was used as a trade item in the earlier days with other tribes and later with white traders (Kehoe 1993).

Horse Days

Once horses and guns were introduced to North America and made their way to Blackfoot society, major changes were introduced. Guns were traded at an early time to the Blackfoot through neighbouring Cree and Assiniboine, who were involved in the fur trade for the Hudson's Bay or the American Fur Companies. Horses were stolen from southern tribes or obtained through an intricate web of trading connections which centred on the Mandan.[11] Horses allowed greater physical mobility, while guns gave superiority over neighbouring tribes and defence of hunting territory. Both interventions had a major impact on how prairie society was shaped. Males as hunters developed strategies that made them more independent of the collective buffalo drives during spring and fall and thus shifted the former balance of equal contribution by both sexes. Men now had more time to spend on ceremonial activities and needed more female labour to process their exploits. This led to a rise of all kinds of military fraternities, the emergence of male-dominated societies emphasizing the warrior as the ideal male image, and changes in the size of families and subsequent role of women.

It is in this period, which began around 1700 and ended with the treaty days around 1875, that the first major encounters with white men took place. Occasional written and visual records of Peigan appeared (Bodmer, in Wied 1976, Kane 1968, Catlin 1973) and shaped, in the non-Native public eye, the image of the "proud warrior" as the prototype of the Blackfoot Indian.

Early Contact

Although individual white people had met Peigan earlier during the horse days (see Appendix B), the latter experienced the first serious pressures on their land around 1830, when the first whisky traders moved into their territory.[12] This led to the appearance of the NWMP and, in their footsteps, settlers and merchants who provided services for the police. It is during this short period (1830 to 1877) that the Peigan culture began to deteriorate, when traditional social structures started to be challenged, abetted by the introduction of alcohol,[13] when chiefs started losing their influence, when wildlife and buffalo dwindled in numbers, and when a series of epidemics affected the Peigan. At this time, missionaries, soldiers, and government representatives came into contact with the Peigan, most of them with the intent to "civilize" and "pacify" the Blackfoot by moving them to reserves, making room for white settlers and opening the West for "modernization." In 1872, the United States ratified the boundary treaty of 1846 and South and North Peigan were discouraged from crossing the border, a move that finalized their separation.

Treaty Days

On September 22, 1877, Treaty 7 was signed at Blackfoot Crossing by several chiefs of the Blackfoot, with Sitting on Eagle Tail as the head chief for the North Peigan. Two years later, the buffalo had disappeared and the Peigan were starving. Many left for Montana, believing buffalo were still to be found there, and others tried to live near settlements or moved to the reservation, where they expected to find promised provisions.[14] At this time of confusion, individual and collective breakdown, and hunger, the Canadian government was totally unprepared to implement the promises they had made with the signing of Treaty 7.[15] Instead, it reacted by implementing a series of interventions, with the Indian agent as the kingpin in this enterprise.[16] Each reserve had an agent who made all decisions[17] and was in charge of handing out jobs. Missionaries started small day schools[18] and made the first attempts to help the Peigan with health problems. Ranch instructors started the first agricultural and ranching activities, but all economic development was under the auspices of the Indian agents.

The Early Twentieth Century

By the beginning of the twentieth century, the Peigan population had declined sharply and many of the traditional Peigan social institutions seemed to have vanished. The knowledgeable older people had died, the middle-aged residents struggled for survival and had little time for ceremonial activities, and agents and missionaries applied various strategies to change their "wards" from "backward heathens" to progressive ranchers and farmers. This was done by undermining or forbidding any kind of religious activity[19] and by putting children into residential schools.[20]

Any training beyond the primary grades happened in so-called industrial schools for students between the ages of fourteen and eighteen. These were usually off reserve and taught various trades to boys and household skills to girls.

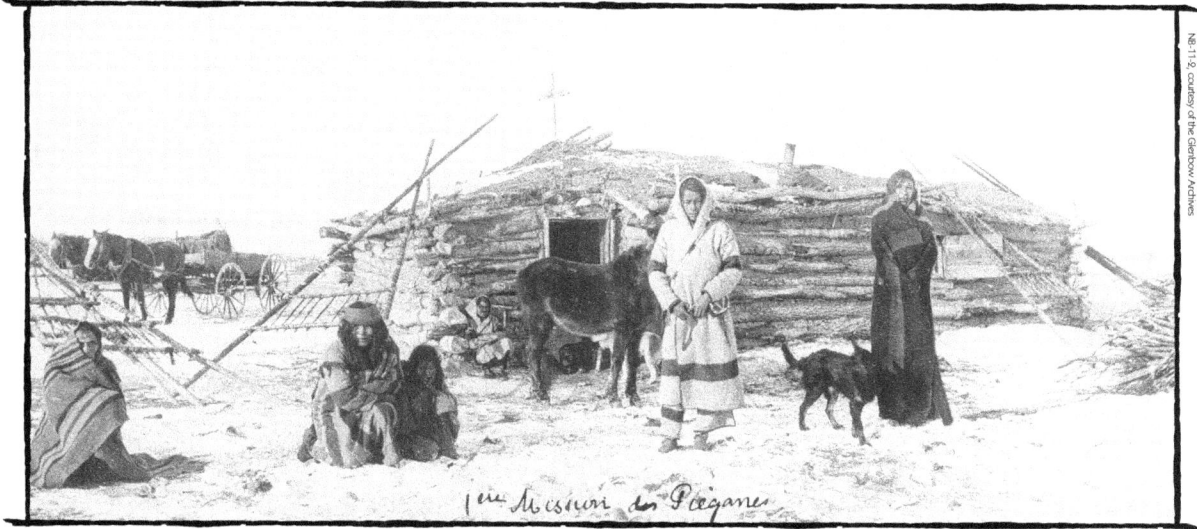

First Catholic mission on Peigan reserve, Alberta, [ca. 1880s].

Dunbow School south of Calgary was the boarding school attended by most Peigan children who went on in education. North Axe, former head chief of the North Peigan, was one of the first students to attend.[21]

In the beginning of the twentieth century, the Department of Indian Affairs set up teaching farms and hired farming and ranching instructors. But often supplies and equipment were not available or were substandard. In the Treaty 7 area, in 1894, the government offered cattle in exchange for horses. But North Peigan efforts towards self-sufficiency were again subject to government intervention. Based on the pressure of land-hungry settlers and political and economic interests in getting the West settled (for example, those of Canadian Pacific Railway Company), Ottawa in 1909 forced a vote on the North Peigan to sell 28,496 acres of their surveyed reserve land, a process that was also imposed on other Treaty 7 nations (Doucet, no date).

Population

Although we have only limited data on how health was perceived in the days before the treaty was signed, certain other information can be used to deduce the health of the Peigan people. Health status is based on factors such as population size and changes, impact of epidemics, and periods of starvation.

In 1801, Alexander McKenzie estimated all members of the Blackfoot tribes at 9,000 (Berry 1953), while Dempsey (1986) gave for 1823 a figure for all Blackfoot of 11,200, the Peigan alone numbering 4,200. Catlin (1973) gave a figure of 16,500 souls in 1832 for all Blackfoot tribes, and Maximilian zu Wied (1976) in 1834 estimated all three tribes as 18,000 to 20,000 people strong. Another estimate by Dempsey (1986) in 1841 puts all Blackfoot at 6,350 and the North Peigan at 2,500. Hind estimated the figure at 7,600 in 1858 (Berry 1953). But in 1869 all Blackfoot were again at 9,216, and the North Peigan had grown to 3,960 people (Dempsey 1986). In 1870, another estimate put the Blackfoot (including the American division of the Peigan) at 13,200, with the total Peigan population at 4,400 (Turner 1950). In 1882, there were about 6,500 Natives

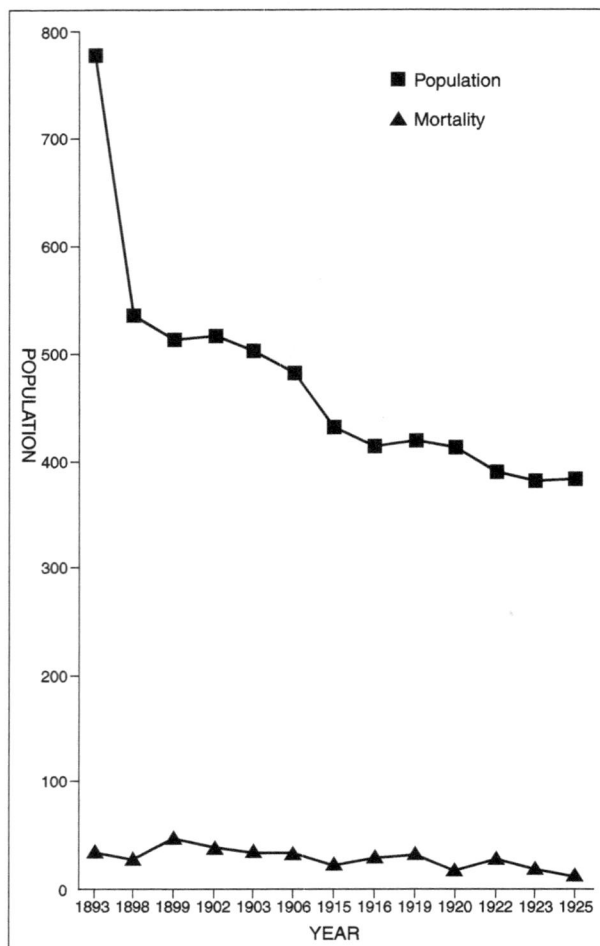

Graph 1. Population and mortality
of the North Peigan

on all three Canadian reserves, with about 4,000 on the Blood and North Peigan (Turner 1950). In 1884, the total Peigan population was estimated to be about 4,000 strong, with 1,000 living in Canada as North Peigan (Dunn 1994).

Another figure in 1885 counts the Canadian Blackfoot tribes at 5,380, with the North Peigan at 929 members (Gray 1971). Another count by Haydon (Hale 1885) in 1885 reports all Canadian Blackfoot at 6,000, with the Canadian Peigan at 800 and the American Peigan at 2,300. In 1888, the North Peigan population was placed at 932,

and, by 1909, there were only 471 North Peigan left (Samek 1987). Doucet (no date) gives for the years 1909, 1910, and 1911 the figures of 471, 416, and 448, respectively. In 1948, Canadian Blackfoot numbered 3,584, but for the North Peigan, only 635 (Berry 1953).

Although some early counts are based on estimates,[22] there is a pattern visible that clearly shows times of population stress for all Blackfoot, Peigan, and the North Peigan in particular (see graph 2).

Treaty payment ledgers for the Peigan reserve covering the period between 1893 and 1936 (Oldman River Culture Centre) give additional evidence of the population size of the North Peigan (see graph 1). However, these numbers cannot be seen as absolute as, in the early reservation days, many North Peigan would not have registered with the agency on the Peigan reserve, or might not have given the correct number for their family members, as this would have affected the amount of ration distributed.

Starvation

Although early descriptions and images of the Blackfoot people give the impression of a relatively healthy population, wintercounts are one of the sources mentioning periods of starvation, which must have had an impact on population size.[23]

The Bull Plume wintercount (Raczka 1979) mentions the years of 1825 and 1861 as ones of starvation.[24] The Bad Head wintercount gives 1854 as the time "when we ate dogs"; the only other time mentioned is 1879 to 1881 "when the buffalo disappeared." Running Rabbit's wintercount gives 1883 as the time they were "eating dogs." McClintock (1935) gives 1877 as a starvation year.

Other, non-Native sources mention as lean years the period between 1879 and 1881 (Dunn 1994, Potyondi 1992), and even up to 1886, when hundreds[25] of Blackfoot died of starvation (Higinbotham 1978).[26]

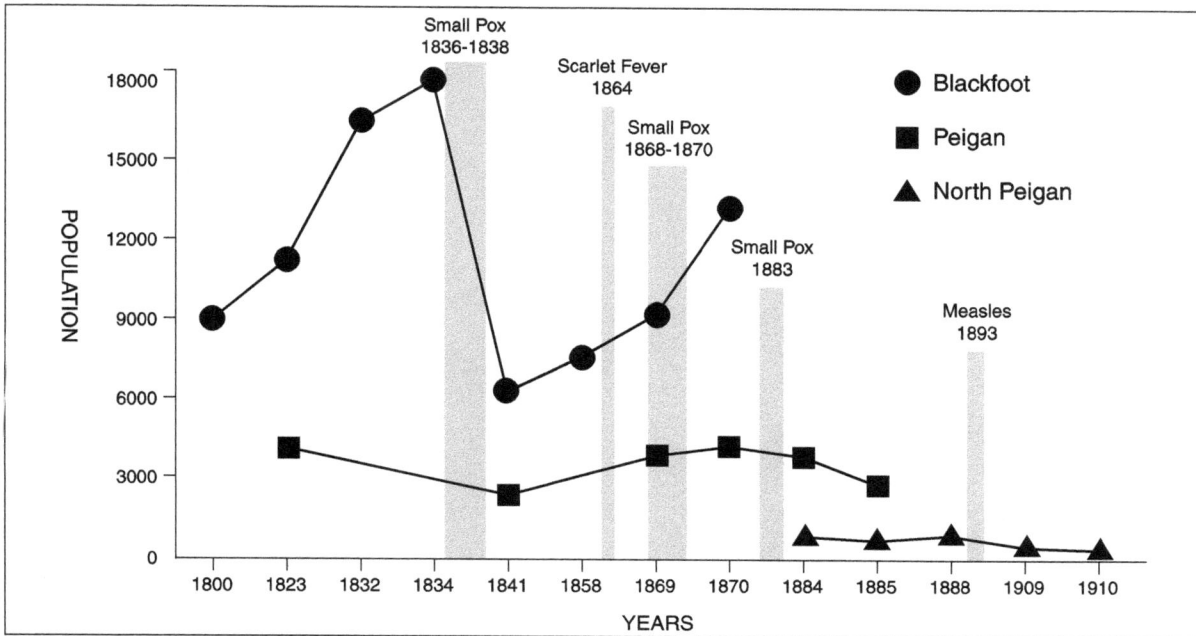

Graph 2. Epidemics affecting populations of Blackfoot, Peigan, and North Peigan.

Epidemics

Bull Plume's wintercount (Raczka 1979) mentions that smallpox reached the Peigan in 1764 (although Raczka believes this was the 1781 epidemic), and cough disease in 1780. The next major smallpox epidemic recorded is in 1837, and, in 1864, scarlet fever reached the Peigan. Another smaller smallpox epidemic happened in 1868, and 1883 is called the Year of Disease. In 1893, children died from measles. Bad Head (Dempsey 1965) reports a coughing epidemic and measles in 1819, the first smallpox from 1837 to 1838, scarlet fever in 1864, and smallpox again in 1869 to 1870. Running Rabbit's manuscript notes smallpox in 1868, 1893, and 1897 and blackpox (black measles or scarlet fever) in 1873.

MacGregor (1949) reports smallpox outbreaks in the Saskatchewan area in 1735, 1781, 1816, 1856, and again in 1870. Although the epidemic is reported for areas on the fringes of Blackfoot territory, there is reason to believe that the disease might also have affected the three tribes. In fact, Thompson's informant, Saukamappee, mentions in 1781 a smallpox outbreak that happened some

years back when his tribe was travelling. The year 1781 is also mentioned by other authors as the time when the Peigan contracted smallpox after attacking a Shoshoni (Snake Indian) camp; the epidemic resulted in the death of half of the Blackfoot (Dempsey 1986). Another epidemic in 1836 killed two-thirds of the Blackfoot.

A smallpox epidemic in 1867 to 1870 killed, in Reverend McDougall's estimation, about 675 Blackfoot, 1,080 Peigan, and 630 Bloods (Dunn 1994). Berry (1953) reports a smallpox plague within the Blackfoot Confederacy in 1869 that killed about 1,400 men. Steele (1915) mentions an outbreak from 1870 to 1877 that affected all Plains Indians, including the Blackfoot people.

Dempsey (1986) notes that the Blackfoot experienced a smallpox epidemic after 1841 and another one in 1870. In 1890, a flu epidemic killed adults, including North Axe, the head chief of the North Peigan, and many children. In 1894, a measles epidemic killed about thirty children and was followed by another outbreak in 1901.

Thus various epidemics, mainly smallpox, measles, and, in later years, tuberculosis had a major effect on the health of the Peigan population.

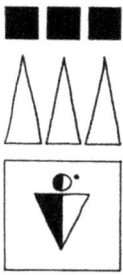

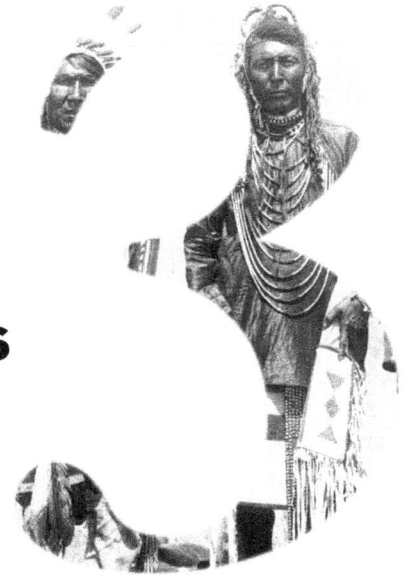

Social Structures

This chapter describes how the Peigan/Blackfoot people organized themselves and related to each other and contains a discussion of social roles and institutions. The most significant groups were, and to some extent still are, the family, extended family (kindred), band, tribal group, and societies.

Family and Extended Family

As far as can be reconstructed, at the time of contact, a family usually consisted of all the family members living in one lodge: the male head of the household, his wife or wives, and their children. Sometimes, this small group was joined by an older relative who could not live by her/himself or a young male relative who was "raised" by the head of the household and was his helper.

Traditionally, the parents of the future bride and groom arranged the marriages, and gifts were exchanged between the two families once an agreement was reached.[1] The bride's family usually provided the new household, which included a new tipi with furnishings. Once the tipi was set up next to the groom's father's lodge, the new couple moved in and started a family. If the bride was not the first wife of her husband, she would move into her husband's tipi and have a separate sleeping place.[2] Although a young couple's tipi was usually set up next to tipis belonging to the husband's family, sometimes a husband would move the couple's tipi to his wife's relative's camp. This was particularly the case when he was one of many sons and his wife's parents had no sons of their own.

The "head" of this bigger group of several tipis would be the oldest male in the central household; for example, the father of the groom. A settlement thus consisted of a man's tipi with his wives and his children, his sons and their families in their lodges, and a few relatives. Children were often raised by their grandparents or other family members rather than their biological parents, and formal adoptions were frequent. Such an extended family was based on co-operation to survive, with clear role definitions for each member. At the same time, this arrangement allowed for a certain amount of privacy for the members and individual families.

There were certain attributes attached to "good families," reflected by the abilities of the men and women to be good providers as hunters and gatherers, the women's contributions as housekeepers, and the possession of certain properties, such as horses. Normally, the oldest members of a family had the most respected positions, another indicator emphasizing the importance of seniority in Peigan/Blackfoot culture. Children were regarded as belonging to a father's family, and a woman divorced her husband by moving back to her parent's tipi. If her parents were dead, she would move back to her brother's or kin's lodge.

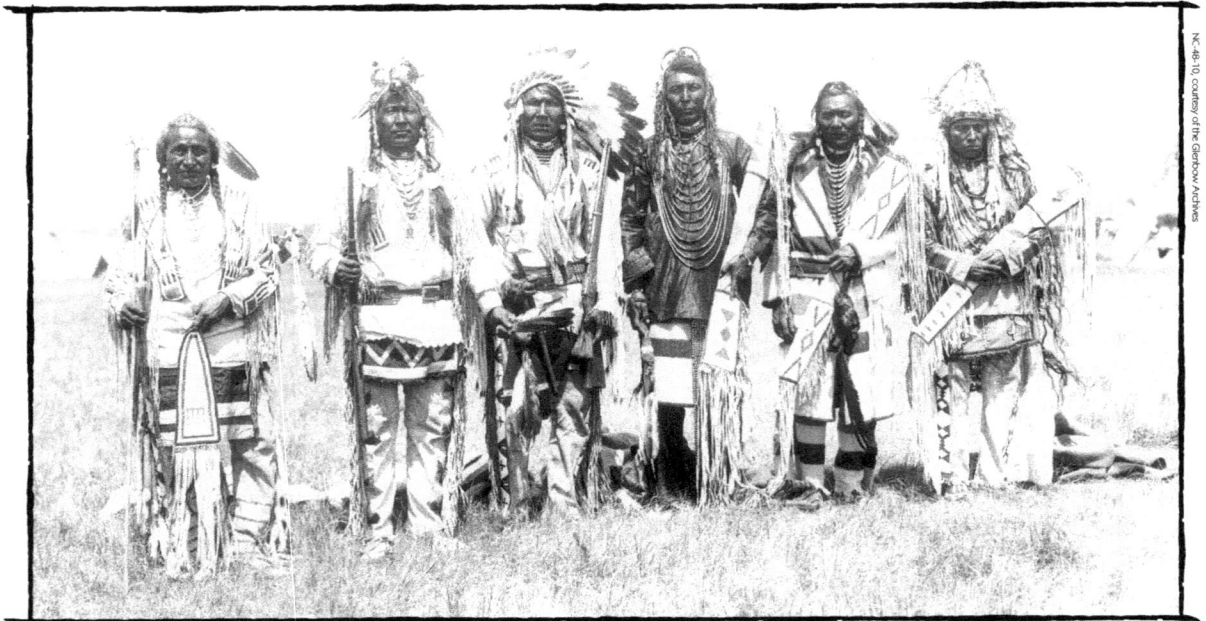

Traditional Blackfoot All Brave Dog Society

Bands

Bands[3] were not just residential groups of extended family members, but comprised several groups of people who were all relatives of an individual's maternal or paternal lineage. Members belonged to their father's band, and marriage between members of the same band was in most cases prohibited.[4] They customarily camped together all year round and accepted one older male in their group as the leader. Bands were flexible enough to move easily for hunting and gathering, but at the same time were large enough to defend themselves from enemies. Kehoe (1993) argues that about one hundred individuals were necessary to conduct successful bison drives, which included "20 to 40 active men and a similar number of active women. This size reflects the number of adults required to construct and man the corral and process sufficient of the slaughter herd to support the community for a few weeks....The 'raison d'être' for the community is the operation of the drive, in a sense, the band is the task group" (p. 93). As a man was related to several chiefs, through his own

or his wife's lineage, he could decide to change bands whenever he wished and move to another camp. Thus, an extended family could split off and form its own, new band[5] or join another band, but this move was not taken lightly.

Historical information on band names by Native and non-Native sources is neither conclusive nor complete. Most information pertains to the Blackfeet (Grinnell 1892, Uhlenbeck 1911, Wissler 1910) or Blood (Hanks and Hanks 1950, Haydon 1971, Morgan 1964), and little data were obtained from the North Peigan. Sully (1870) mentions two band names: the Strangulated (Eka-tapis-tax), with One that Sees Before (Zoa-pia) as chief, and the People of the Lake (Omak-siki-nutapi), with the Northern Chief (Apo-to-sina) as leader, counting 32 and 28 lodges and 384 and 336, members, respectively. Grinnell (1892) mentions three bands: Seldom-Lonesome, Dried Meat, and No Parfleche.[6] Emile Legal (1885), one of the first Oblate missionaries living with the North Peigan, names seven different bands: Dried Meat, Many Pains, Red Excrements, Homeless or Blood People, Women with Black Chest, Those Who Fight Alone, and Sorcerers. Raczka (1979) suggests:

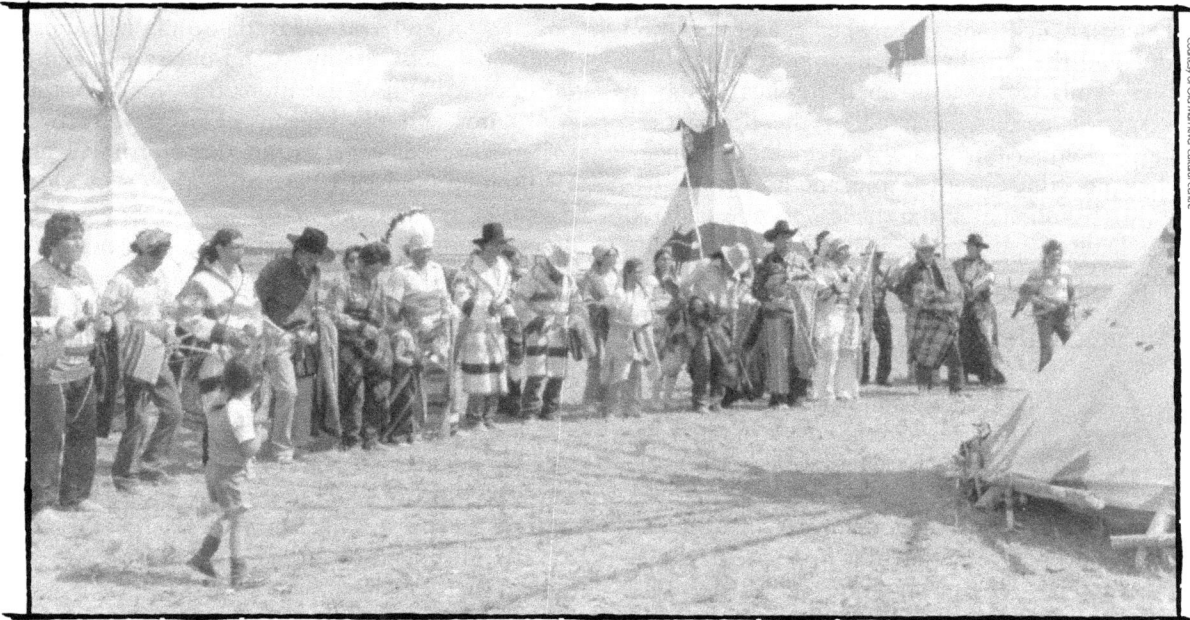

Courtesy of Old Man River Cultural Centre

Modern Peigan All Brave Dog Society

...six recognized bands among the North Peigan. They are the Seldom-Lonesome (Miawachpitsi), Gopher-eaters (Omachkokatauyi), White-Breasts (Axichokimix), Blood or Bullrush People (Apaitapix), Hairy-Nose or Padded-Saddles (Imoyiskistsi or Kutsakiita) and Lone-Fighters (Nitaikskaiks). The Seldom-Lonesomes have three sub-bands, the Never-Laughs (Katayiimix), Coyote-Cut-Bank (Mahkoyo-isatako) and the White-Robes (Ksiksikokas). The new names for the Seldom-Lonesome came about due to camping locations on the reserve. The Lone-Fighters were evidently low on numbers at one point in their history and were joined by members of the northern division of the Greasemelters. It should be pointed out that bands did not name themselves but were given names according to their habits or characteristics observed by other bands (p. 9).

Bands also received names based on specific characteristics of their leaders or an attribute related to a certain historic incident. They were like nicknames and could change when they became out-dated or a new incident occurred. Given this constant fluctuation of band affiliation, the period of time when these names were known and reported gives evidence of important events that affected Blackfoot culture. Warfare, epidemics, and starvation had effects on population size and thus on new or decreasing numbers of bands.[7] Additionally, the signing of the treaties led to the replacement of traditional chiefs, outstanding men of dominant extended family groups who were often former warriors and advisors with agent-appointed band members.[8]

In their study of the Blood, Hanks and Hanks (1950) observed that the band as an organizational unit had disappeared but that most families still lived in house clusters of extended family groups.

Tribe

Several bands coming together would form a tribe. During most of the year, band camps were scattered over their traditional lands, but once a year all bands came together to meet in the tribal camp. This was during the central ceremony, the Okan (Sun

Dance), which took place when the berries were ripe and the buffalo concentrated in large numbers. Tipis were set up in the annual camp in a specific pattern, dictated by the tipi owners' band membership. Regular members set up on the outer fringes of the camp, and leaders of societies, ceremonialists, and the leaders of each band would pitch their tipis in concentric circles around the centre.

Societies

A Blackfoot person would belong to various societies in the course of his or her life. These societies were essential to the survival of the whole tribe and were not kin-based but reflected an individual's interest and personality. Societies usually had specific functions and had leaders who were identified by specific paraphernalia and were regarded as chiefs. Military societies were related to fighting but additionally had internal policing functions. Nearly all of these societies were age-graded. Thus, a young man started out joining the Bees, then became a member of the Mosquitos, and worked his way through different ranks until he was a member of the Brave Dogs, the Horns, or the Old Bulls. Because of these memberships in different societies, new ties to members outside of one's own biological ties and social circles were established. These new relationships were also built on mutual support. In pre-reservation days, all tribal members belonged to one or several different societies and thus had numerous kinship connections with people in their own generation. Because of the reduction of the population and the decreased interest in traditional aspects of Blackfoot culture, many societies disappeared.[9]

In 1833, on his expedition up the Missouri River, Maximilian zu Wied (1905) observed dances by certain societies: the Mosquitoes (young boys between eight and ten years of age with young men as leaders), the Dogs (young married men), the Prairie Dogs (policing society for married men), Those Who Carry the Raven (policing society), the Buffalo (helpers of the soldiers), the Soldiers (most distinguished warriors,

policing society), and the Buffalo Bulls (the most distinguished of all unions and oldest and highest in rank). Wilson mentions that, in 1893, the Mosquitos and the Pigeons (Doves) were two societies in existence within the North Peigan (Wilson, in Godsell 1958). Since the reservation days (i.e., from about 1920), a young boy might enter one of his father's or uncle's societies and eventually move from one age-graded subsection to the next. For example, he might, with the help of his relatives, join the Crazy Dog society, and, in the following years, move through different stages of membership until he became a leader.

Nick Smith (no date), a Peigan elder, remembers the following societies: the Black Horse society, the Skinny Black Horse society, the Red Coat society, the Brave Dog society, and the Piegan society. The last two are newer societies with a more social mandate. At present, on the Peigan reserve, there exist the Black Horse, the Red Coat, and the Crazy Dogs societies. The most long-lasting are the Brave Dogs or Crazy Dogs (Knut-some-taix). They were regarded as having great power because they were composed of past chiefs who had earned a reputation for bravery and strictness. They were known to kill men who refused to obey orders. They policed the tribal ceremonies and hunts and worked with the tribal government to enforce law and government decisions. They ruled the camp and helped the chiefs to administer public discipline.[10]

Most societies were male fraternities, but all male members needed to have a female partner, a wife, sister, female cousin, or other relative. The Peigan had no exclusively female societies like the Buffalo Women Society of the Blood.

Leadership

L eaders of the military societies had the obligation to protect their camps from enemy attacks and were regarded as chiefs, as they had control of all situations pertaining to policing, hunting, and moving camp. If a society leader showed ongoing qualities of wisdom, good judgment, and bravery, he could become the leader of his tribe. "All bands recognized peace or civil chiefs" (Maclean 1893), and these were responsible for all issues within their band at times when there was no danger from enemies. They presided over council meetings and were responsible for resolving conflicts and hosting important official visitors from other bands. "The civil chief controlled the destiny of his people only so long as the strength of his personality and the obvious correctness of his judgment seemed to indicate his authority" (Lancaster 1966, p. 179). Usually, one of these leaders was identified as head chief and would decide, with other leaders, on specific issues like the signing of treaties.[11]

A leader was dependent upon his family's or band's support and had to ensure that all his followers were taken care of. Thus, a chief had to be generous to the less fortunate and sometimes was quite poor himself, as he was obliged to give his material wealth to others. "No Blackfoot can aspire to be looked upon as a head man unless he is able to entertain well, often invite others to his board, and make a practice of relieving the wants of the less fortunate band members" (Wissler 1910, p. 23). Since the reservation days, this system of mutual dependence has changed, as chiefs are elected and are not judged on the basis of the same characteristics as in the past. Now, they have become arms of the federal government and its administration.

Roles of Men and Women

Blackfoot society in the pre-reservation days was centred on males—fathers, uncles, brothers, and other male relatives and members of one's society. These men were clear role models for the boys. However, due to hunting and warfare, father figures were frequently absent, and mothers and (paternal) aunts were primarily responsible for the upbringing of small children. Mothers and fathers were strict with their children, but it was the mother who was in charge of educating and training her daughter as a future wife and lodge keeper.[12]

Still, a person's security and status depended on the performance of his or her male relatives, although Lewis (1941) describes certain women,

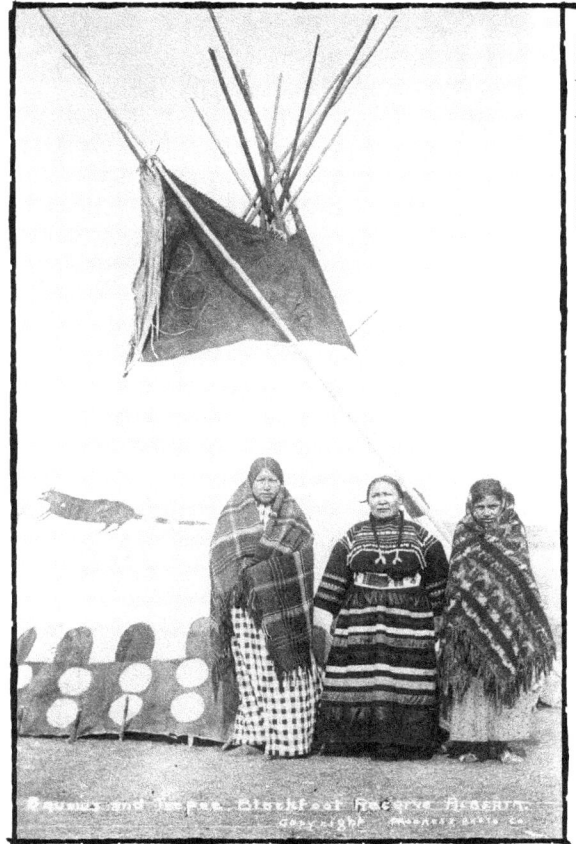

NA 1370-4, courtesy of the Glenbow Archives

Wealthy Peigan women

belonging to the wealthier families, who defied these rigid role expectations and became "manly-hearted" in their ways. However, the majority of Blackfoot women seemed to have followed normal role expectations. First historical records by fur traders and explorers (e.g., Fidler in 1792 and Maximilian zu Wied in 1834) describe them as hard workers who were in charge of all basic chores to ensure the welfare of their camp (Fidler 1991). Male activities centred on hunting and warfare, with the emphasis being on the latter in the form of horse raids on enemy tribes in the period when the first whites came into contact with the Blackfoot people.

A boy's goal in life was to become a good hunter and warrior and eventually a leader of his people; a woman's goal centred on being married to a successful man, having children, and keeping a lodge. Although women were important as suppliers of knowledge and gatherers of food staples, these activities seemed to have been of lesser importance in the historical period of the horse days.

Marriages were polygynous. Women were severely punished, mutilated, or even killed for adultery.[13]

Both men and women had important ritual roles in ceremonies, and women were central players in the Okan (Sun Dance) and partners in some of the more important societies and as bundle owners. But information on women's ceremonial activities around the turn of the century shows that in the horse days ceremonial activities had a tendency to emphasize male participation.[14] Even in the ceremonial context, only a virtuous woman who had been faithful to her husband held prestigious positions and responsibilities in regard to society offices or sacred bundles.[15]

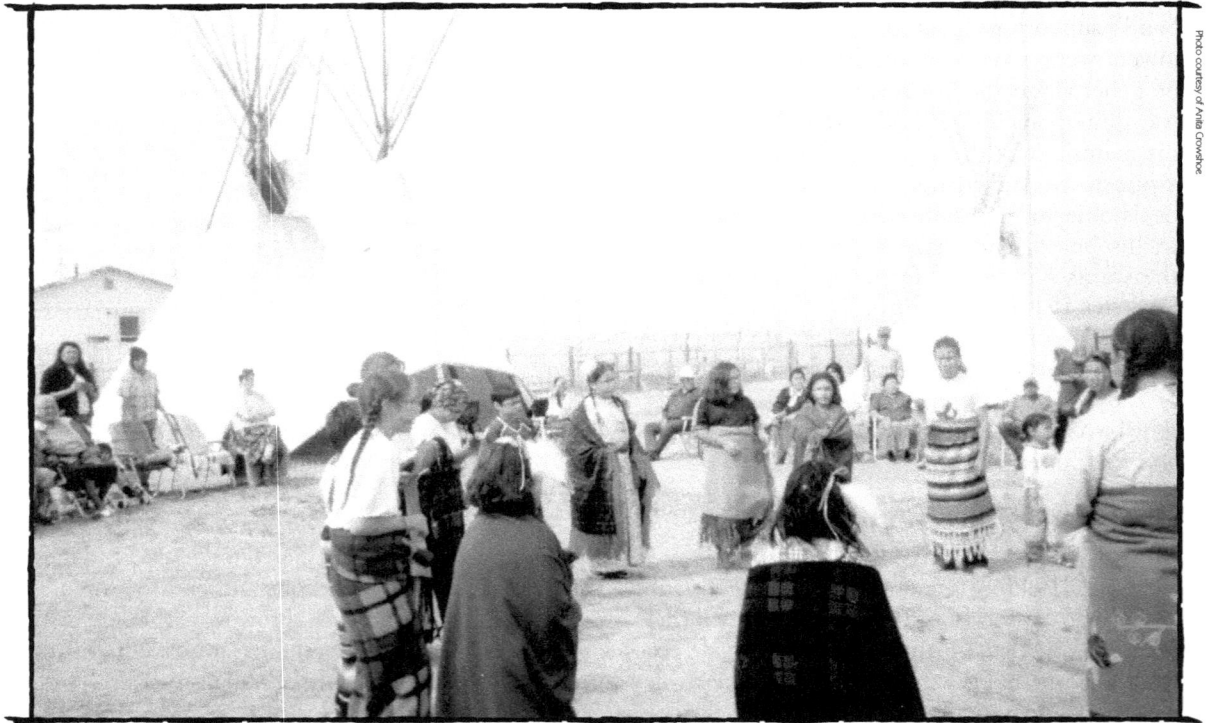

Photo courtesy of Arita Crowshoe

Niipoomaakiiks (Chickadee) Society (8- to 14-year-olds).

Peigan/Blackfoot Concepts of Sacred Bundles and their Functions

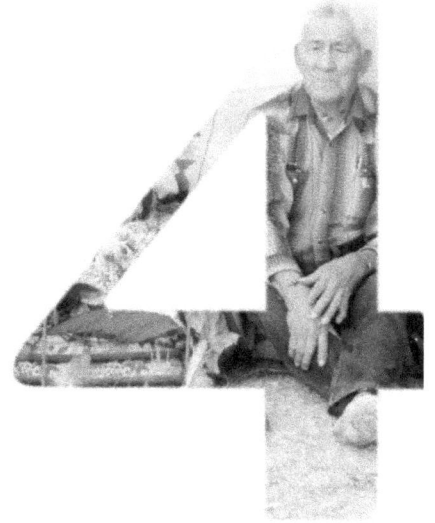

From a traditional perspective on Peigan/Blackfoot culture, ceremonial bundles had and continue to have a central position. These bundles are objects of varying sizes that contain articles that are regarded as sacred.

Bundles ensure the survival and well-being of the community, bands, extended families, and individuals. They also emphasize a person's status, have particular functions, and are the physical and abstract manifestation of the traditional Blackfoot belief and social system.[1] The origins of all bundles are based on an individual's communication with a Creator or a Creator's messengers through a vision involving specific instructions regarding the physical and abstract components of a bundle. Therefore, animals and natural phenomena (like thunder) have physical representations that are part of the bundle's contents. The abstract elements of the bundles are the songs and prayers that are essential to all ceremonial procedures.[2]

There exist a variety of categories of ceremonial and individual bundles, which have particular functions and which need, in order to be used actively, a male and female custodian (or, for the personal bundles, an individual) who will commit themselves to the proper ways of taking care of the particular bundle. Peigan/Blackfoot culture recognizes Sun Dance bundles, Thunder Medicine Pipe bundles, Beaver bundles, various society bundles, and smaller personal bundles. They all vary in size and content and can be transferred from one set of bundle keepers to the next in a particular ceremony.[3]

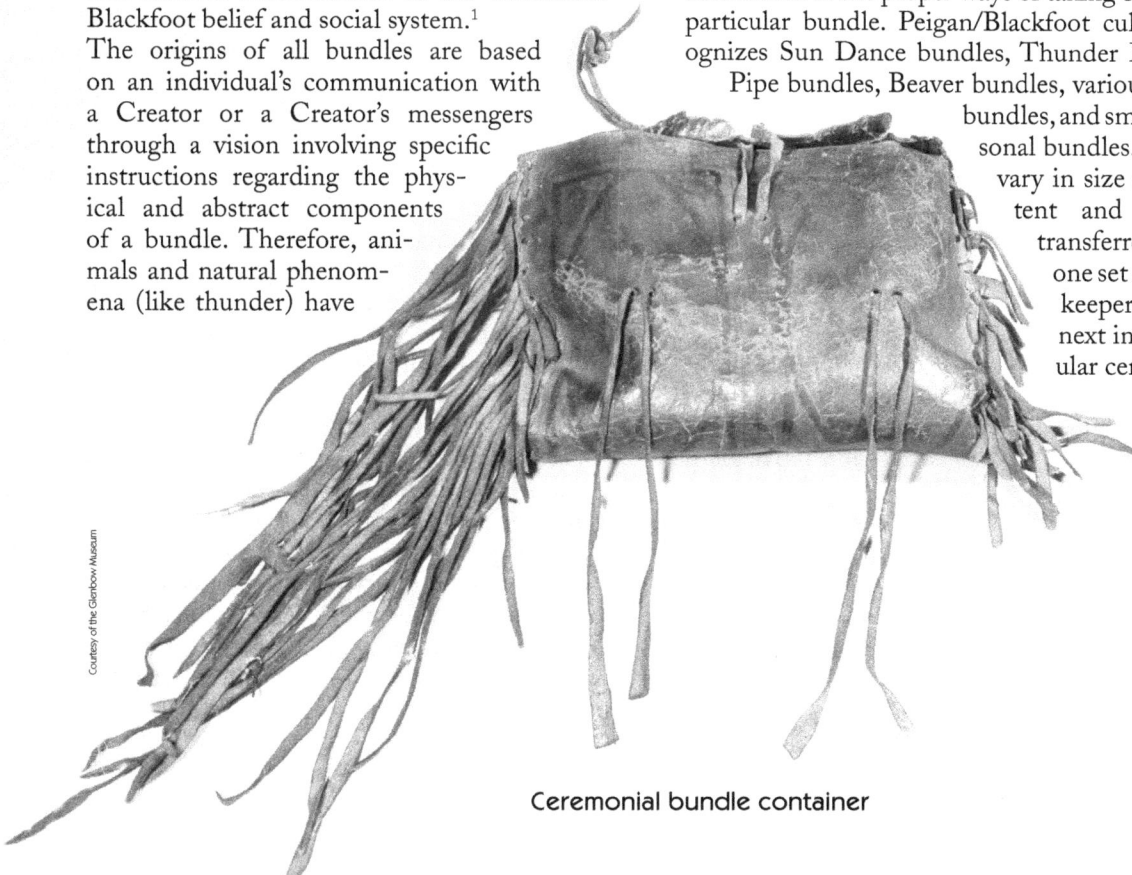

Ceremonial bundle container

Custodians of ceremonial bundles have high status in their communities and are today regarded respectfully as elders. Along with the social benefits of taking care of such a bundle, bundle keepers accept weighty responsibilities by being knowledge-carriers and ensuring, through ongoing ceremonial practice, the well-being of their community.

The following four principles are central to Peigan/Blackfoot traditional ceremonies:

1. Each ceremony has a certain number of cultural materials represented in a bundle that emphasize the bundle's specific function,
2. All ceremonies have two leaders (a man and a woman who are regarded as bundle keepers) who have gone through the proper process of learning the ceremonial procedures (transfer rites),
3. Each ceremony has to be supported by individuals who hold particular functions in relation to the bundle,
4. The ceremonial process has a specific beginning and end, and a protocol defines the appropriate position and duties of each individual participating in the ceremony, as well as the role of the cultural materials involved, namely, the bundle itself, the pipe, and the smudge.

The following text describes all categories of bundles in light of their social and ceremonial functions. Each bundle contains specific objects that are central to its function and role.

The Natoas (Sun Dance Bundle)

This ceremonial bundle is the central object for the successful completion of the Okan (Sun Dance) ceremony. It is primarily a woman's bundle in the sense that it is a Blackfoot female, fulfilling a vow she made at an earlier time, who goes through the Sun Dance ceremony[4] and receives the sacred bundle[5] during its course. The central objects of the Sun Dance bundle are the Holy Woman's headdress, the turnip digger, and the elk hide robe. The origin story of the Natoas is told by various authors and relates primarily to the story of The-Woman-who-Married-a-Star. In McClintock's account (1968), based on Brings-Down-the-Sun's narrative in 1896, Feather Woman is the first to receive the Sun Dance headdress. She marries Morning Star and lives for a while in the sky with her husband and his parents, the Sun and the Moon. Eventually, she returns to her people with her son, Scarface, clothed in an elk hide and with the Natoas headdress and the digging stick.[6] Wissler and Duvall (1995) and Wissler (1912) describe a somewhat different origin story based on the elk woman's seduction by and elopement with an elk other than her husband.[7] Wissler claims that the Natoas bundle was at one time part of the Beaver bundle, as the headdress was worn by the wife of the Beaver bundle owner, who received it from the elk man. He states that, before the presentation of this gift by the elk man, "Scarface brought down the custom of wearing a headband of juniper for the medicine woman, and it is the tradition that this was displaced by the natoas" (Wissler 1912, p. 214).[8] The Sun Dance woman later borrowed the Natoas from the Beaver bundle and eventually purchased it from the owner, thus instigating the development of a separate ceremonial bundle.[9]

In terms of the abstract components of the Sun Dance ceremony, the songs and prayers show great similarity to those of the Beaver bundle ceremonial. But the paintings on the altar and on the body of the Holy Woman's companion show the strong connection with the Morning Star/Mistaken Morning Star origin complex. They, next to Sun and Moon, are the central figures in Blackfoot mythology, and one can assume that, for this reason, the Sun Dance bundle can claim a central position independent from the Beaver bundle.

The social function of the Natoas bundle can be clearly understood by the way in which it was celebrated by all members of the tribe during the summer, when buffalo hunting was not practiced,[10] the berries were ripe, and time for social gathering was necessary. Historical as well as archeological records show that various bands would gather together at a given date in a specific location. They would use this time for social exchanges—settling feuds and conflicts, making marriage arrangements and forming other alliances, giving names, and establishing new allies. Healing ceremonies ranging from individual performances to collective ones, with an emphasis on preventive and general health concerns, played a major role during the Sun Dance.

This ceremony thus offered an umbrella for all kinds of other individual or group activities, as the unifying ritual for the tribal collective rather than only the kinship group or band. The Holy Woman's sacrifice[11] to the Sun, her vow made for the betterment of the tribal community and the insurance of its survival, and the symbolic integration of the planetary constellation's importance into the ceremony are all factors that make the Natoas ceremony the central annual event in a Blackfoot tribe's cycle.[12] The ceremony's function of re-balancing all misgivings between humans, Creation, and Creator and to re-establishing harmony beyond earthly considerations puts it in a superior (or sovereign) position over other ceremonies. In other terms, the Holy Woman's sacrifice with the help of the Sun Dance bundle can restore balance when there is a health problem, when there is a conflict between people themselves or people and the environment, and when there is a lack of buffalo.

The Beaver bundle and the Thunder Medicine Pipe bundle are, after the Natoas, the two bundles of greatest importance to the Blackfoot people. Only Blackfoot members with outstanding leadership characteristics owned these bundles.

The Beaver Bundle

Beaver bundles are also called Tobacco bundles (Fraser, no date) Water Pipe bundles (Schultz 1930), or Water bundles.

Several sets of stories relate to the origins of the Beaver bundle. One of the most detailed accounts comes from McClintock (1968), who, in 1896, visited Mad Wolf, a Beaver man of the Southern Peigan, and gives detailed descriptions of the Beaver bundle ceremonial that he observed in 1906. As told by Mad Wolf, the bundle was brought to the Blackfeet by a young unmarried man called Akaiyan (Old Robe or Round-Cut-Robe), who survived one winter inside a beaver lodge (dam). He returned to his people with the knowledge of the prayers, songs, dances, and the ceremony itself. He also knew how to use roots and herbs, how to treat sickness, and how to mark time.[13] Akayan received instructions on how to build this bundle, with the emphasis of its function of restoring health to the sick or dying. He and the Old Beaver's son stayed in the Blackfeet camp to teach the songs, prayers, and dances. Finally, in the spring, they invited all the animals "to add their power to the Beaver Medicine." Upon the return of the little beaver to his father, Akaiyan received a pipe to add to the bundle. While the origin story strongly emphasizes the bundle's powers of individual healing, the bundle opening and its contents stress its powers to aid the people's physical survival.[14]

Wissler and Duvall (1995) give four versions of the origin of the Beaver medicine, as collected by Duvall between 1902 and 1905. The South Peigan version tells the story of a woman and a young boy who are drowning while attempting to cross the Yellowstone River but get pulled into a beaver's lodge. Although other water animals want to kill them, the beaver takes pity on them and saves their lives. The beaver gives the woman songs and tells her that she will have great powers and live a long life.[15] The Northern Peigan story tells of a married woman who goes to live with the beavers and, upon her return, brings back a large bundle because the beavers pity her. The woman's husband, in a series of dreams, receives instructions for the ceremony and the songs, for the woman's headdress and elk hide, and makes a vow to give the Sun Dance. Tobacco is kept in the bundle and is planted every year by the woman who puts on the headdress and carries the digging stick. In the Blood version, a man and his wife camp at the shores of a lake and the woman goes to the home of the beaver. After some time, she returns to her husband and gives birth to a beaver child. Eventually, the beaver man gives the husband some of his medicine songs and comes to the couple's lodge. He sings a song with the skin of various birds and puts them all together in a bundle. In the Northern Blackfoot version, a wife goes to a lake and comes back with instructions on how her husband will obtain the Beaver bundle. The Sun and Moon come down to lead the ceremony, and all water creatures are present. The Sun gives the songs to the man, and, after four nights of singing, the Beaver bundle is given to the man with instructions to open it in the spring and perform the tobacco planting ceremony.

As told by McLaughlin (1970), the Beaver bundle was obtained by a young man called Api-Kunni. He was poor, had no relations, and was badly clothed. In order to gain the love of a young woman, he decided to go on the warpath. Wandering through the prairies, he fell asleep on a beaver house, and the beavers took him in. They kept him through the winter and taught him many things. Before he left in the spring to go on the warpath, they gave him war medicine and instructions. He killed an enemy with the power of the beaver medicine, scalped the man, and counted coup. Upon returning to the camp, he became chief and married his girl. He taught the people what the beavers had told him, including the planting and use of tobacco.

It is not mentioned when this last story was collected, who the author used as informant, and to which tribal subdivision this story pertains. But the two other reports, by Wissler and Duvall and McClintock, respectively, explain the Beaver bundle as a gift or payment given by the Underwater People. The Beaver man, therefore, has power over water and can revive the drowned and control the weather.[16] He is also regarded as a weather forecaster. He has the power to call the buffalo and ask other animals for help. He keeps track of time, and thus develops outstanding oratory skills and becomes the "memory bank" of his people's history. The Beaver man would remember information on good springs and waterholes in specific geographic areas, on patterns of movements of certain animals, and the like.[17] The Beaver bundle helps a band or a group of people to make daily decisions regarding local survival.

In September 1965, the Provincial Museum of Alberta purchased the Calling-Last Beaver bundle from its owner, a resident of the Blood reserve. During the ceremony, a participant, Albert Chief Calf, told the story how he was protected by this specific "water bundle" when he was young and in a skirmish with a white man from Calgary, who shot at him. This confirms the Beaver bundle's additional function as a potent protection in war.

The Thunder Medicine Pipe Bundle

As the name reveals, these types of bundles are related to thunder, and the origin story identifies thunder as the power that gave the pipe to the first owner in a vision.[18] This vision included instructions on how to create such a bundle, what the individual parts of the bundle had to be, what handling process had to be followed, and what kind of taboos went with the bundle. The central object in the bundle is the Medicine Pipe, but there are other objects that have been added to the bundle. These include specific animals and their hides, as well as buffalo stones and rattles. The drums that are used to accompany the songs and dances in the ceremonies are also specific to the Medicine Pipe bundles, as their sound represents thunder.

Bodmer, the painter who travelled with the German prince Maximilian zu Wied, was the first to depict a Blackfoot Medicine Pipe.[19] There exists a series of photographs of Thunder Pipes and bundles in the works of McClintock (1968) and Wissler (1941), which were taken around the turn of the twentieth century.

Origin stories about Thunder Pipes have been published by several authors, notably, Wissler and Duvall (1995) and McClintock (1968). The latter relates the story of Brings-Down-the-Sun or Running Wolf, whose father Iron Shirt went near the summit of Chief Mountain and there met Thunder Maker, who appeared in the form of a bird. Listening to the instructions of the Thunder Bird, Iron Shirt made a pipe and added it to his bundle. This pipe was a Long Time Pipe and was smoked only on important occasions.[20] Wissler and Duvall's information comes from the Blood and tells the story of a girl who married

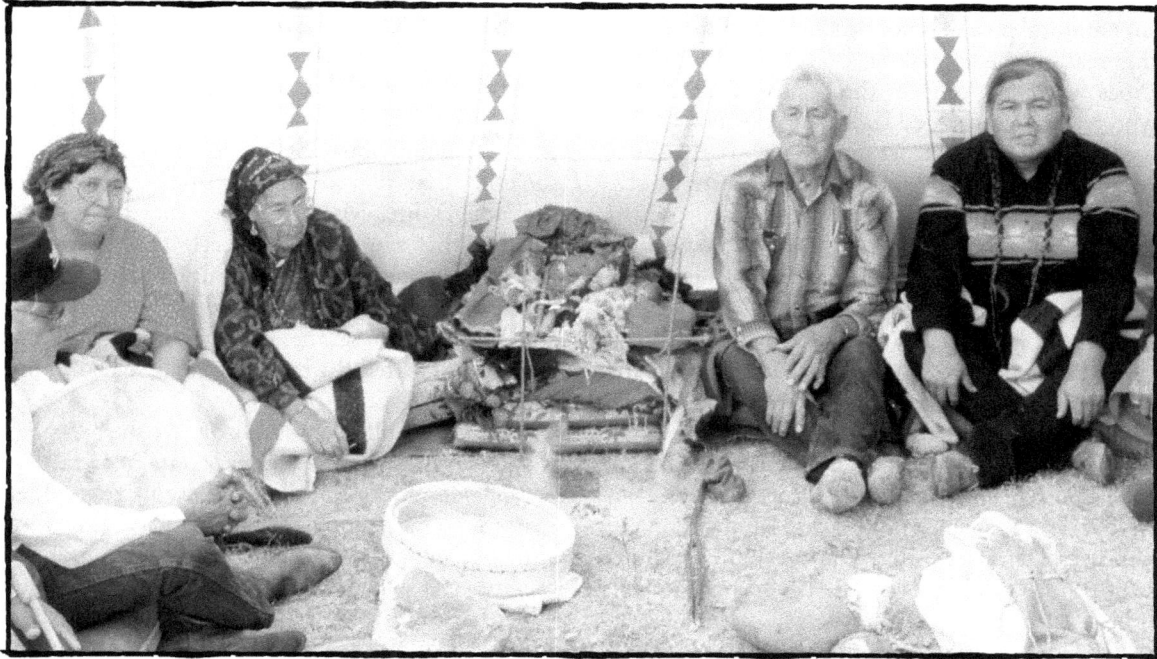

Peigan Thunder Medicine Pipe bundle (Left to right: Floyd Rider, Rosemary Crowshoe, Molly Kickingwoman, George Kickingwoman, and Reg Crowshoe).

Thunder and brought the pipe bundle back on a visit to her people. Thunder accompanied her and transferred the pipe to the members of her family.[21] Dempsey (1962) interviewed Steve Oka, a Blood resident, on the origin of the Thunder Pipe bundle and was told:

Its origin is common to all medicine pipe bundles in that it was supposed to have been given by the Thunder to a man who successfully defied him. Thunder stole a man's wife and took her to his lodge. When they arrived he removed her eyes and hung them from a string, together with numerous other eyes that he had obtained. The husband followed for many weeks until he met a raven, who directed him to Thunder's lodge. He gave the man certain powers so that he was able to defy Thunder and successfully identify his wife's eyes. Before he left, he became friends with Thunder and was given the medicine pipe bundle (p. 74).

As with the other ceremonial bundles, a man who wanted to receive a Thunder Pipe was to go into an isolated place and, exposed to the sun by altitude, after many days of fasting and praying, receive instructions in a dream or a vision. In the case of the Thunder Pipe, the messenger could be a supernatural being or an animal, primarily powerful ones like the buffalo, beaver, wolf, grizzly bear, or eagle. But often helpers were personified natural forces like Thunder, Wind, Storm, and Blizzard. The person looking to attain such a pipe did this either for personal reasons or to gain knowledge to help his or her community.

The function of the Thunder Pipe relates to its supernatural power and strength, its ability to decide over life and death and thus heal people from certain sicknesses. Additionally, Thunder Pipes are used to settle conflicts and disputes between individuals or groups of people.[22] Any offence against an agreement settled with the smoking of these pipes was regarded as a severe violation that would be punished through death by a supernatural power, if not by Thunder himself. For this reason, the caretaking of Thunder Medicine Pipes was often only in the hands of older men who had acknowledged leadership positions.[23]

Although there exist a variety of Thunder Medicine Pipes and bundles, which were mostly named after a specific characteristic of the pipe or its origin, it is the Long Time Pipe Medicine bundles that have unique significance. Others were called Rider Medicine Pipe bundles or Mounted Medicine Pipe bundles (the owner had to ride on a certain horse),[24] Sits Backwards or Opposite Pipe Medicine Pipe bundles, Little or Short Medicine Pipe bundles, and "Captured" Medicine Pipe bundles (for example, the Gros Ventre Medicine Pipe, the Cree Medicine Pipe, the Eastern Man Medicine Pipe, and Chippewa Medicine Pipe bundles [Dempsey 1962, David Melting Tallow 1966]). Joe Gambler from the Bloods explains:

> Red Crow owned the Long Time Pipe, only the head chiefs will purchase the Long Time Pipe. In the past before the white man came the head chiefs are the ones that will own the Long Time Pipe. Times went by and when Owns Many Horses became head chief he took the Long Time Pipe. When he died his son Crop Eared Wolf also became the head chief and he took the Long Time Pipe, it's the rich people that purchase the Long Time Pipe. Gambler (1968)

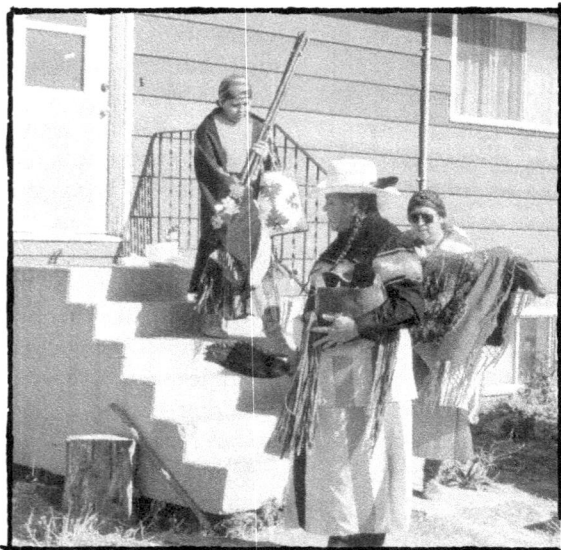

Co-author Reg Crowshoe and family leaving for ceremony.

Societies' Bundles

As described in Chapter 3, Blackfoot culture was very structured, and each individual belonged to one or more societies that played an important part in the individual's life. Many of these societies owned bundles that symbolized the role they played in Blackfoot society. Societies gained their "right" to form themselves from dreams or a vision, and often in these the material items and the songs that created the bundle were revealed to the dreamer.

The Old Bulls were advisors to the younger warriors, and their bundles contained rattles. Membership in this society was exclusive to older males who had a long track-record of being wise and courageous leaders. The Seizor's or Catcher's society consisted of middle-aged males who had enough authority (based on their war deeds) to demand that others fulfill specific requests for the leaders. The main item in their medicine bundle was a pipe, which was regarded as potent war medicine (Wildschut, 1912). The first owner of this pipe bundle was camped near the present-day Head-Smashed-In Buffalo Jump and was a buffalo caller.[25] The Brave Dog or Crazy Dog society had policing functions; their bundle contained rattles and a couple of bear headdresses and belts that were handed out to individuals who had leadership roles in this society. The Prairie Chicken, Pigeon, and Bumblebee societies all had a defined role to play in Peigan society and special objects to symbolize this role, which were wrapped in a bundle.

The present-day Horns and Buffalo Women (Motokiks) societies have a strong role and use their own bundles in their ceremonies. Some Peigan reserve residents are members in these societies. However, the Blood were primarily active in these societies, which did not seem to have a role in historic Peigan culture.

All of the previously mentioned bundles, when handed over to the care of another society member, need to go through a transfer ceremony in many ways similar to the process mentioned earlier. David Melting Tallow (1966) includes in his list of transferable items the following society bundles: four Horn bundles, two Motokiks bundles, three Crazy Dogs bundles, one Prairie Chicken bundle, one Pigeon bundle, one Crow Carriers bundle, and one All Braves bundle. All society bundles mentioned are in relation to the Blood tribe. This list is not exclusive but most likely mentions all the society bundles that were still in use at the beginning of this century.

Individual or Personal Bundles

A personal bundle was an object that was regarded as sacred and therefore powerful and had a special function for its carrier. It served as protection from sickness, starvation, bad weather, and drowning; from being caught by the enemy,[26] and to ensure old age. Smaller objects often included necklaces and wristlets, which were regarded as personal protection and worn either all the time or for particular occasions.[27] But there were other personal bundles that an individual could use to help others in matters of life and survival.

Among the most common and oldest personal bundles are *iniskims* or buffalo stones, specially shaped rocks in animal or human form, often parts of ammonites. They are also found in Beaver and Thunder Pipe bundles but can be regarded as individual bundles in themselves. They are essential for the calling of the buffalo, especially in times of hunger or starvation. The origin story tells of the woman who brings the special stone into her tipi.[28] Although Wissler (1912) calls some big rock formations *iniskim*, this name seems to have been primarily applied to the smaller rocks, which were moved around. Other smaller bundles were medicinal or herbal bundles, tipi bundles, and tipi flag bundles, shields, headdresses, shirts, and bear knives; but there were also bigger ones like the Black Tail Deer, the Feather Game, and the Hand Game bundle. David Melting Tallow (1966) lists individual bundles that need to be transferred: the child's topknot and head band, holy robes, tipi designs, tipi flags, buckskin suits, war bonnets, war shirts, dance whips, ghost dance headpiece, deer dance headpiece, war shields, big

drums, shaman's curing bundle, and holy hand-game bundles.

Although all personal bundles enhanced or ensured the well-being of their wearer or owner, some gave the individual additional powers to heal or cure others. For example, a personal healing kit, purchased by the Glenbow Museum, was primarily used for treatment of pneumonia.[29] Birth control bundles were used to help women avoid pregnancies.[30] Another object fitting into this category is the Little Beaver Skin bundle, which a series of famous Blackfoot medicine men used to cure people and whose powers were also received in a dream by its first owner Came from Above (Dempsey 1961).

Bigger bundles, like most Horse Medicine bundles, embrace a whole ceremonial complex and have to hang on a tripod.[31] Their function is to help cure horses, but they are also used as protection for people going to war or on a trip or expedition. In addition to its veterinarian function, it also helps to increase the speed of race horses. The Black Tail Deer bundle is also one of the bigger personal bundles that is used for curing the sick. The bundle and its ceremony were first introduced to the South Peigan by the Kootenais, probably at the end of the nineteenth century. McClintock (1969) mentions that it is made to charm game, making the capture of deer easy due to the hunter's hypnotic powers, and gives the hunter speed and endurance.

In conclusion, one can state that the small medicine bundles (in the nature of personal charms or fetishes, personal war and curing bundles) were of foremost interest to their owner, as they ensured his or her personal survival and protection. They were often buried with their owners and were seldom handed on. Then there were bigger bundles, regarded as personal with specific benefits bestowed on the individual owner. These were handed down from generation to generation and could help others in a very specific way. Sometimes, additions based on dreams were made to these bundles, and then the bundle evolved, acquiring a more complex ritual that entailed the participation of other individuals, and thus developed into a more esteemed bundle. The society bundles, then, had very particular functions in their community. The Thunder Pipe specialized in resolving conflicts between individuals or groups of people, ensuring goodwill and cooperation, thus serving a critical function in the survival of the Blackfoot people. The function of the Beaver bundle principally related to local survival, based on the knowledge harboured in both the bundle and the owner. It helped a select group of people, a band or extended family or even a tribe. It had all the information pertaining to the group's local survival, which meant knowledge about time and geography and animal behaviours and patterns. The Natoas bundle served to ensure the survival of the whole Blackfoot tribe by re-establishing a balance among all parts of Creation and the Creator.

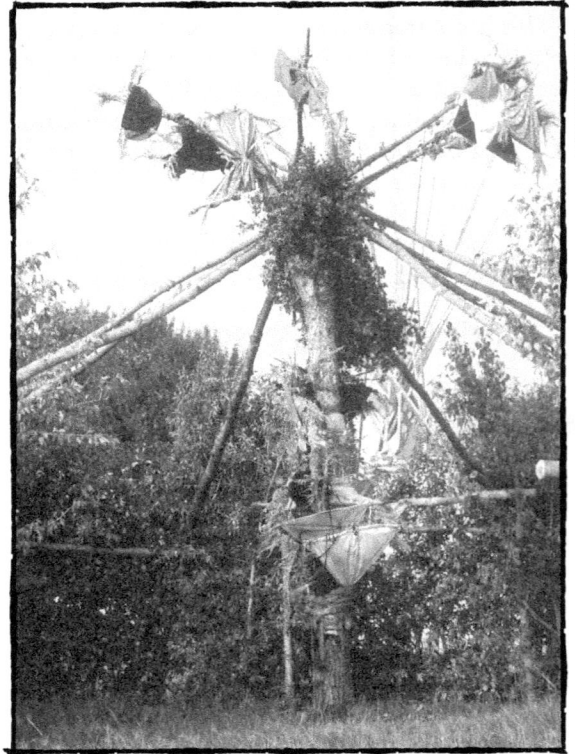

Centre Pole of Sun Dance Lodge.

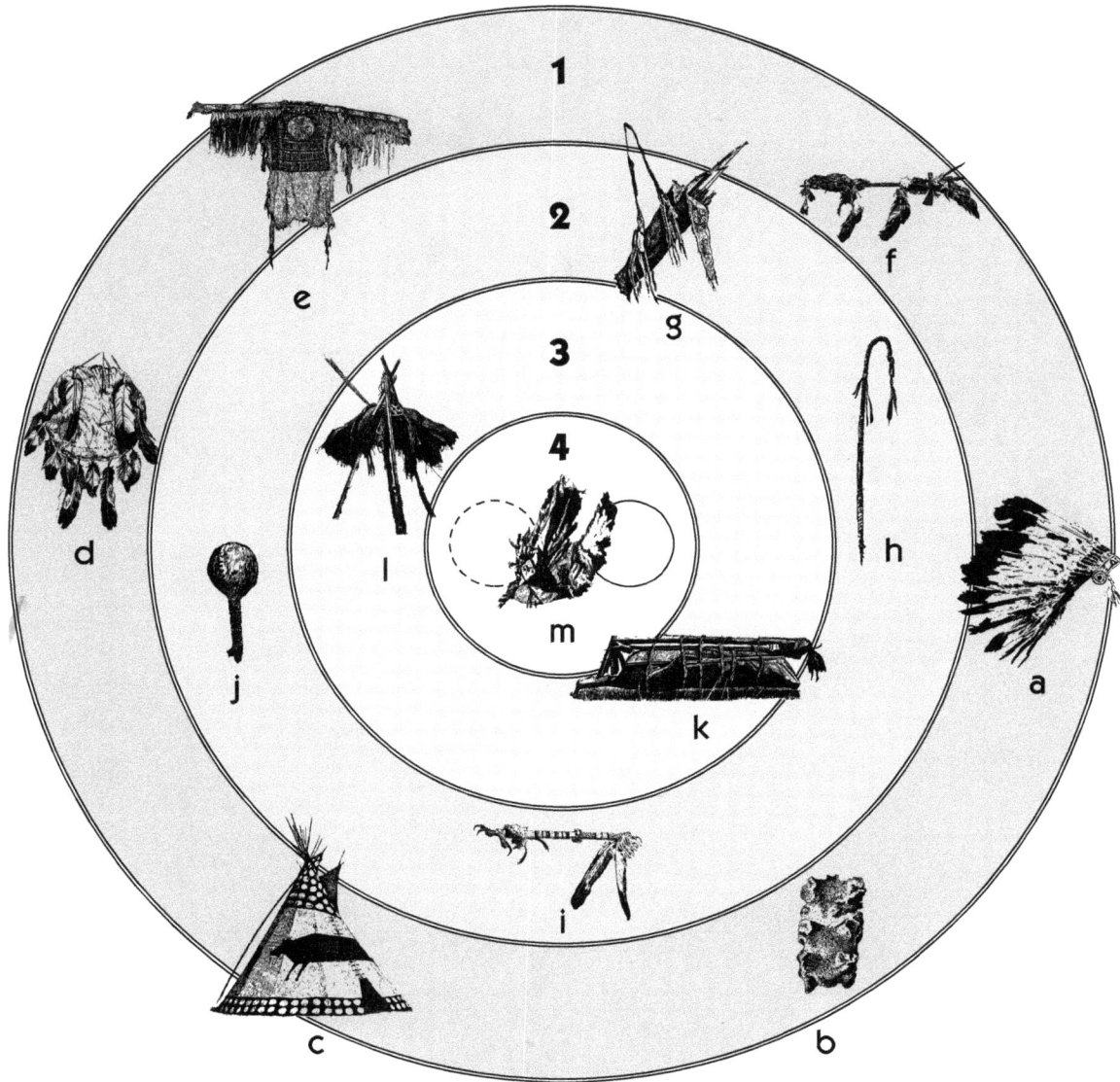

Ring 1: Personal Bundles
  a. Headress
  b. Buffalo Stone
  c. Tipi Design
  d. Shield
  e. Weasel Tail Shirt
  f. Pipe

Ring 2: Societies' Bundles
  g. Bow and Arrow
  h. Staff
  i. Eagle Claw Staff
  j. Rattle

Ring 3: Ceremonial Bundles
  k. Beaver Bundle
  l. Thunder Medicine Pipe

Ring 4: Sovereign Bungle
  m. Natoas Bundle

Transferable Items

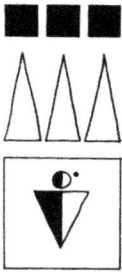

Transfer Rites

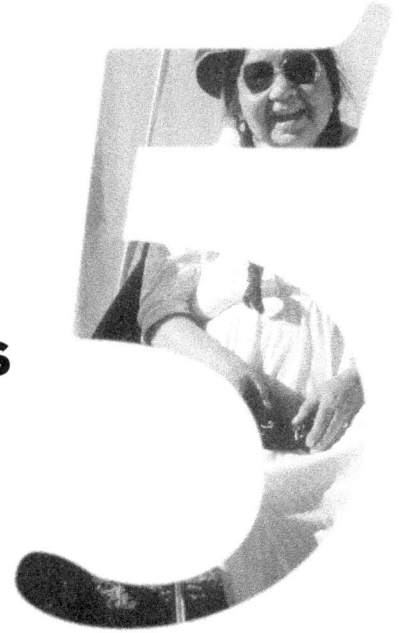

In Blackfoot culture, when a bundle was constructed for the first time or moved from one set of caretakers to the next, or when certain objects were added to or removed from the bundle, a ritual ensured that this process was done in the right way. This ritual was called a transfer rite or ceremony. An individual who wanted to handle, pray with, or take care of sacred objects had to participate in such a transferal.

Originally, all articles regarded as sacred were received through the Creator or one of the Creator's manifestations (for example, Thunder, the Beaver people, or the Elk and other animals). The person was given a dream or vision with instructions to build a sacred object out of specific materials. This process was called *giimmaks'inn*, as the recipient received a gift from the Creator in pity for his or her suffering.

Also, an individual had the option to receive materials and knowledge in payment from an animal or a supernatural being, or to obtain the sacred articles in capture or payment from another person who had received these at an earlier time. In this case, the transfer is called *poomaks'inn*, which describes the process of making a payment for a transfer. Both *giimmaks'inn* and *poomaks'inn* are essential concepts in understanding transfer rites in Blackfoot culture.

A person who had a dream was likely someone with an outstanding reputation[1] who was exposed to a number of ritual experiences. Once he or she decided that the dream had religious significance, respected leaders and other ritualists were invited to the dreamer's lodge. After smoking the pipe, the dreamer told his or her experience and asked witnesses for support. By smoking the pipe, participants indicated that they accepted the dream as truthful and consequently discussed what they would contribute in terms of songs, materials, and prayers. After the initial meeting, the dreamer started making the physical bundle and collecting various items. Finally, the dreamer went through an official transfer ceremony to establish stewardship when his or her face got painted.

However, this process of making a new ceremonial bundle was very rare and was regarded as a highly dangerous endeavour. For example, New Breast, one of Duvall's informants interviewed in 1911, states:

[A] person can make up any sacred bundle or thing when he has a dream to do so. But he must get others to help him who knows some thing about such a bundle or those who has owned such a bundle.... it is very dangerous to make up any sacred bundle when he never was told to do so through a dream or told to do so by some one else.... Bull Child, once asked [New Breast] to help him make up a medicine pipe, but he refused to help him as he knew it was very dangerous. But Bull Child, made a medicine pipe and sold it to Mr Clark Wissler, and soon after he had done so, his wife died and then Bull Child died. It is very dangerous to make up these things without being told to do so by the owners or through a dream. Spotted Eagle made up a Na-to-as, and sold it to a white man, and soon died after he had done so. It is even dangerous to tell lies about these sacred bundles or talk about some sacred bundle that a person has no right to, that is to tell about some thing that he does not own or never owned. (Duvall 1911, pp. 4–5)

Thus, it was rare that a person went through a *giimaks'inn* transfer rite for a major ceremonial bundle. Such people needed to have outstanding self-confidence.

When a person was interested in taking over a major ceremonial object that was owned by someone else, he or she would usually consider a transfer rite by payment or *poomaks'inn*. In this case, the person approached the owner with a pipe that the owner smoked if he or she agreed to hand over the bundle. But if the owner took the pipe and shook out the tobacco or returned it unsmoked, this meant a refusal to give up the bundle. Sometimes, the bundle owner himself

looked for an appropriate candidate. He could inquire indirectly if there was a potential candidate, but his helper could also capture a person, who would then become the new owner. The earliest report on such a capture comes from McClintock (1948), who describes how Wolf Plume was captured by scouts who were sent out by the Medicine Pipe bundle owner.

Ceremonial bundles weren't the only objects to be transferred by payment; any other object that was regarded as sacred (e.g., the weather dancer outfit and the Medicine Pipe Headband and Plume) could be transferred in this way as well (Kipp 1965).[2] Another, more recent, account by First Rider (1974) describes another means of obtaining a ceremonial bundle, by stealing the sacred object:

Now a person admires a medicine pipe and he tries to get it, he is already prepared for what he is going to pay, so he gives for the pipe, he enters the tipi while the people are sound asleep and he steals the medicine pipe, it is actually the rule to steal the medicine pipe.[3]

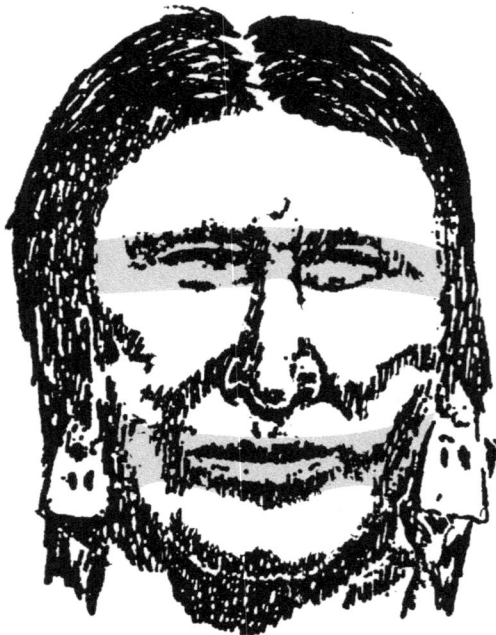

Brave Dog face paint

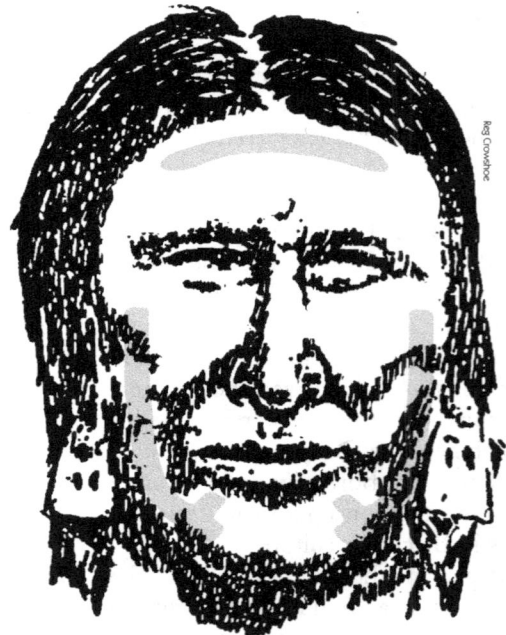

Thunder Medicine Pipe face paint

30

The procedure also varied depending on what kind of sacred object the buyer wanted to obtain and how prestigious it was, but the principles behind each transfer ceremony remain the same. They are: a person can approach another person to get the article; the present owners are willing to transfer; there is an abstract and a physical component that get transferred; there is a group of peers who witness the process; there are former owners present; and the new owner is willing to make the appropriate payment.

By going through a *giimaks'inn* or *poomaks'inn* transfer rite, an individual obtains the rights to use certain abstract and physical manifestations. These are songs, stories, and the handling of the specific sacred material. Although these rights are on some level comparable to Western concepts of copyright law,[4] they come with specific responsibilities. The keepers are responsible for taking care of one of the Creator's gifts and for using this gift for the survival of their community.

The transfer ceremony is a process of certification by peers, which, once achieved, gives the owner specific authority. In that ceremony, the present owner will bestow, with the help of former owners, the abstract authority on the new owner. This is symbolized in the face paint applied, the prayers said, and the songs given and taught to the new owner. In this way, the theoretical or abstract knowledge is transferred with the physical bundle and its contents. Prior to the transfer ceremony, a new owner will have gone through a learning process regarding the abstract and physical aspects of the sacred object. Once the new owner's face is painted and he or she has danced with the material, that person is, under traditional Blackfoot law, the legal owner. The paint gives the owner abstract authority, the material bestows physical authority, and the songs tie both aspects together. The owner then can "rightfully" use these three aspects to help others when they are sick or need support. Only the person who received the paint in a transfer ceremony has the authority to sing these songs. The strictness of these rules is often reflected upon by ceremonialists and owners of sacred items: "When a person receives the paint for any ceremonial object, the object is considered his property and there can't be any dispute over the ownership" (Hellson 1966). Another example concerns the proper transfer of a specific part of a bigger bundle:

> I'll tell you the story why I do the drumming. The deceased Sat-Away-from-Him he was the one that initiated me into drumming. The time when Three Suns transferred his bundle to Pink-Tail-Feathers it was then when I was initiated into drumming and I was made to dance with that pipe. One Gun knows it. My father paid good on it. That is the reason why I sing the medicine pipe songs (Joe Good Eagle, in Melting Tallow 1967).

There are different levels of importance of sacred objects. The more important the object, the more formal the ceremony. Ceremonial bundles need a man and a woman to go through the ceremony at the same time. But the Sun Dance headdress and the Buffalo Women's society bundles have only women owners. War-related materials were owned primarily by men (for example, the Seizor's pipe). Personal or smaller bundles have individual owners, men or women, who go through a simpler ceremony. However, as men take care of the physical side of the ceremony by guiding and running it and the women have the abstract ownership, both sexes need to be present for all the bigger objects.

In the transfer ceremony, the transfer of the power of the bundle is symbolically re-enacted. The old owners address the new owners as their sacred children, and the new owners address the previous owners as their parents. All former owners of the bundle who are present are the "grandparents," whose role it is to conduct the transfer ceremony, to tell the history of the bundle, and to instruct on the daily handling and the taboos that have to be followed. The current owners present the new couple with new clothes (sometimes specific outfits go with specific bundles). This is to confirm their new status as children to their ceremonial parents:

When a medicine pipe bundle or any other holy bundle is transferred to a man and a woman they will be born again spiritually and they will be the children to the man and the woman that transferred their medicine pipe bundle or any other holy bundle to them. (Melting Tallow 1967)

Duvall (1911) calls the buyers of a bundle "son" and "daughter" and the sellers "mother" and "father," and the person who leads the ceremony is called the "transferor." One of his informants is even more specific about the roles each participant has to play in the ceremony:

As a rule, whenever anything in the line of sacred articles are to be transferred, they must always have a third party or six person in all three women and three men. Of course they [*sic*] are a few things such as the weasel tail suits, and a few others which would not require women partners. But nearly all other sacred bundles, lodges and thing, generally all require women partners, and these women are usually the wives of the seller and the buyer and the transferors. Now then suppose the man, who is to buy or sell or transfer the sacred outfit, has no wife. He would have to get some woman to act or be his partner during the transferring ceremony.

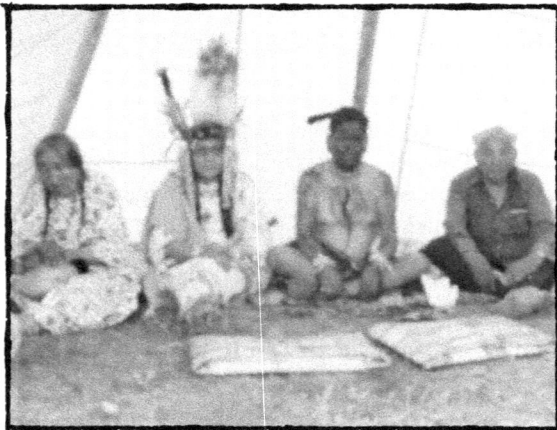

Sundance ceremony (Mrs. Blackplume, Josephine Crowshoe, Joe Crowshoe, Mike Swimsunder).

And of course the woman would also own some interest in the outfit he bought. And the same way with the woman who made a vow to give the Sundance. Should this woman be a single woman she would have to get some of her brothers or uncle or cousins to be her man, partner, during her medicine lodge ceremony. But she would not get any body out side of her own kin folks." (Split Ears, in Duvall 1911)

With high-ranking and certain other society bundles, some individuals can gain part-ownership to specific objects. For example, New Breast tells Duvall (1936) that, in the Natoas transfer, the woman who made the vow has a choice: "She can borrow a Natoas and pay for its use or buy one, but she is more honoured if she buys, but in the olden times these women only borrow it."

The new owner pays the old one with blankets, horses, and other property as an expression of gratitude. The new owner has to be generous, and the old owner can refuse the transfer if he or she is not happy with the payment being offered. Sometimes, the old owner withholds certain parts of a bundle and might be able to create a new bundle with the missing pieces. This explains the many bundles in each category, although at one time there existed only one bundle of each type.

In conclusion, it may be remarked that anyone can make up a natoas, if he has a dream so directing him; also, if he owned a natoas that was lost or otherwise destroyed; if he gave it away, without receiving payment; or if it was buried with someone. Having owned a natoas and transferred it, he cannot duplicate it; should the new owner lose it, he may, if called upon, replace it; likewise, if buried, the surviving husband or wife could call upon him. In all such cases fees are given. When one transfers a medicine bundle and has been paid for it, he has no more right to it and cannot duplicate it on his own motion. Should one sell the bundle without the ceremony of transfer, the ritual remains with him and he can again make up the bundle; should one make the transfer and fail to receive the pay, or waive the pay, he can make it up again. The relatives of one buried with a bundle can call upon a former owner to make it up, after which it must be formally transferred to one of them. Men were sometimes killed on the warpath and their bundles lost; such were replaced as noted above. In every case these must be true duplicates; it is only a dream that authorizes new creation, or variations, however slight. (Wissler 1918, p. 247)

Also, sometimes only the physical part of a bundle was handed on, and in this case the transfer was regarded as incomplete. However, if these were purely personal sacred items and they were handed from family member to family member, there was no need for the presence of other owners, peers, or the public as witnesses.

Thus, although there are some strictly guarded principles to ensure the proper "certification" of the new owners, transfer rites involve a set of rules that guide a ceremonialist's actions. These rules are general guidelines, and it is their interpretation that is essential to the survival of these sacred objects over generations and periods of cultural change. An example is the integration of horses into the cultural complex of ceremonial bundles.[5] Again, in the old bundles, whistles were wooden; and later, whistles made out of gunbarrel were added. However, in all cases, the songs, dances, prayers, and paint used are the same.

Although the process of a transfer ritual is in all aspects clearly defined in Blackfoot traditional culture,[6] confusion begins when unauthorized persons take over the role of ceremonial grandparents or parents to new owners, or when people without "certification" claim to have obtained transfer rites.[7] Consequently, many people who have not been raised in the proper traditions are confused over what counts as a formal ceremonial authorization and what is informal and can be utilized by the general public.[8] For example, sweats can be used by anybody like a sauna or just for cleansing. But a healing sweat can only be conducted by someone who has received transfer rites in the physical form of a tipi design, an individual sacred bundle that might be part of a society or a ceremonial bundle.[9]

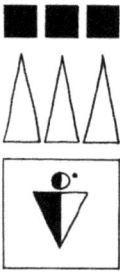

The Blackfoot Circle Structure Process

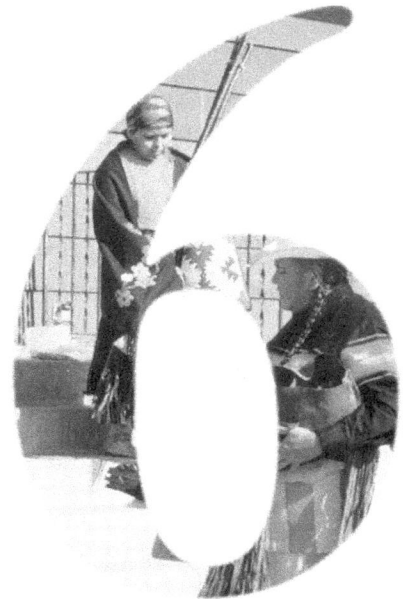

The Blackfoot Circle Structure is a specific model in the physical format following a tipi (circular) floor plan and a process based on traditional Blackfoot ceremonies.

Traditional ceremonies took place in tipis over hundreds of years and many generations, and there exist various descriptions of these rituals. Additionally, Wissler (1913), with the help of Duvall, had his Blackfeet informants draw sketches of various society ceremonies. The sketch of the Pigeon society ceremony indicates the positions of leaders and drummers, the sketch on the ceremony of the Braves shows drummers, leaders, and different categories of members, and the diagram of the Buffalo Women's society ceremony gives even more detailed information on positions and roles of participants and cultural materials.

This text uses and analyzes these graphics as well as the textual descriptions, oral records of still-living ceremonialists, and observations of present-day ceremonial practices. Four guiding principles were identified as being central to all:

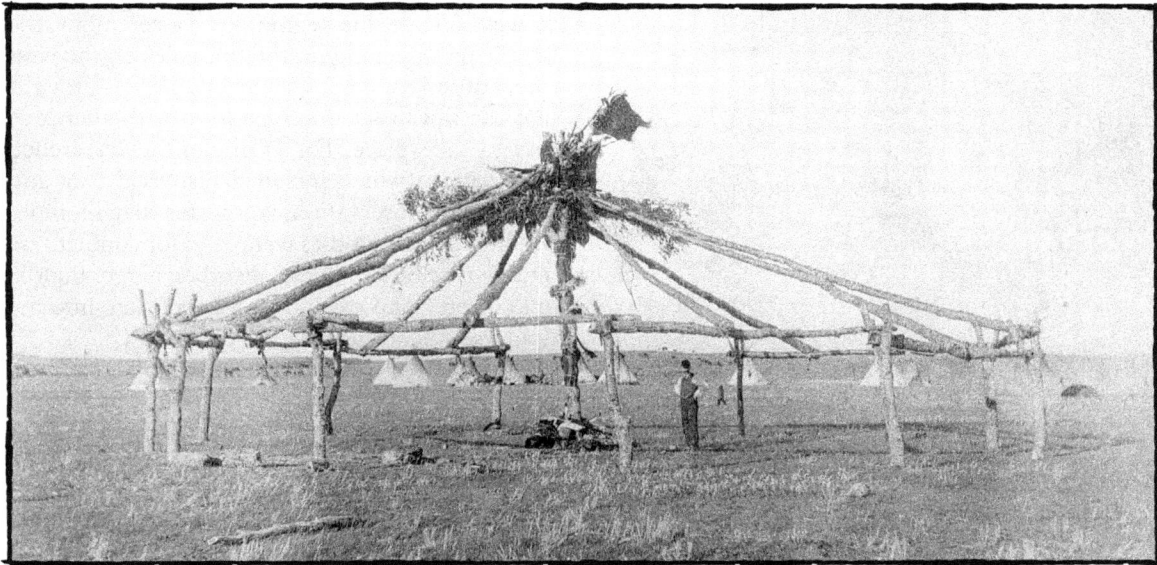

Sundance lodge circle structure.

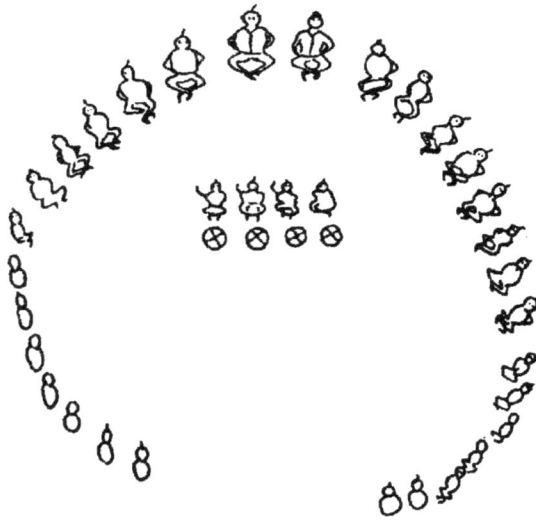

Source: Wissler, 1913

Sketch drawn by a Peigan showing the position of the Pigeon society in a ceremony.

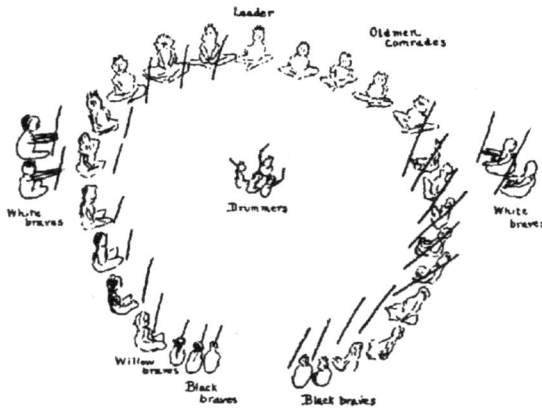

Source: Wissler, 1913

Sketch showing the positions of the Braves in a ceremony.

1. each ceremony had a certain amount of cultural materials represented in a bundle;
2. all ceremonies had two leaders and two hosts (a man and a woman who were former bundle keepers and a man and a woman who were present stewards of a bundle);
3. each ceremony had to be supported by individuals who held particular functions in relation to the bundle; and
4. there was a particular ceremonial process in place that had a specific beginning and ending, and a particular protocol that defined the appropriate position and duties of each individual participating in the ceremony, as well as the role of the cultural materials involved, namely, the bundle itself, the pipe, and the smudge.

Every ceremony took place in the shape of a circle, facilitated by the floor plan of the tipi. The entrance always opened to the east, and the most sacred or important objects were situated inside the tipi on the west side. In all Blackfoot ceremonies, the women sat on the left or south side and the men on the right or north side. A fireplace was dug into the center, and an altar was built on its west side. In the beginning of a ceremony, the bundle usually hung on the tipi poles on the west side, but sometimes a specific bundle was brought into the tipi to set the stage for a particular process to take place. For example, the researched information (which included historical data and present-day observations) indicates that Thunder Medicine Pipe bundles were used for conflict resolution. For other issues, any other, bigger bundle or a society bundle could have been taken into the tipi to set the agenda for the ceremony.

All bundles had a male and female steward, both initiated ceremonialists who had gone through a ceremony of transfer rites and thus had the expertise to handle and take care of one of these bundles. Additionally, there were older, former bundle keepers,[1] who had the role of guiding the ceremony. They were the man and woman sitting on the left and right side of the bundle, respectively, and they were responsible for taking the bundle down and unwrapping and handling all parts of it. These two ceremonialists led the prayers and started the songs in the ceremony and played key roles in guiding the process.

Each ceremony had other participants who took part in the ritual. These were other bundle owners and members or leaders of various societies. Women and men were equal participants in these ceremonies but had specific roles and seating positions. The fireplace at the centre of the tipi was attended to by a man who also served as helper and tobacco cutter to the ceremonialist leading the ceremony. This helper had also gone through transfer rites for this responsibility. He had two additional helpers who brought in firewood, served tea, and assisted in any other matter. On the south side of the tipi, sitting in front of the women, were usually four drummers who were directed by the ceremonialists to sing the appropriate songs during the ritual process. Bundle protocol required that each object be danced with by other bundle owners. The drummers' responsibility was to sing the songs according to the objects. Near the tipi door, older ceremonialists and former bundle owners took their seat. They had the role of observing the proceedings and making sure that everything was done in the right order and that the ceremonial protocol was adhered to. Additionally, they represented the continuity and importance of this traditional worldview.

The beginning of a ceremony was signified with a smudge. Smudging is the placing of hot coals on an altar and the burning of sweet pine needles or pieces of sweetgrass on the hot coals.[2] The ending was symbolized with the smoking of a pipe, either a secondary pipe that was part of a bundle or a special pipe that the bundle keeper used for these occasions.

These descriptions of historical bundle ceremonies correspond exactly to rituals that take place in present-day Blackfoot communities. It is this ceremonial process that has been translated for Western applications or practices and thus is used as a model for decision-making processes in modern Peigan life.

The tipi floor plan, with specific positions and roles for participants, shapes the ceremonial

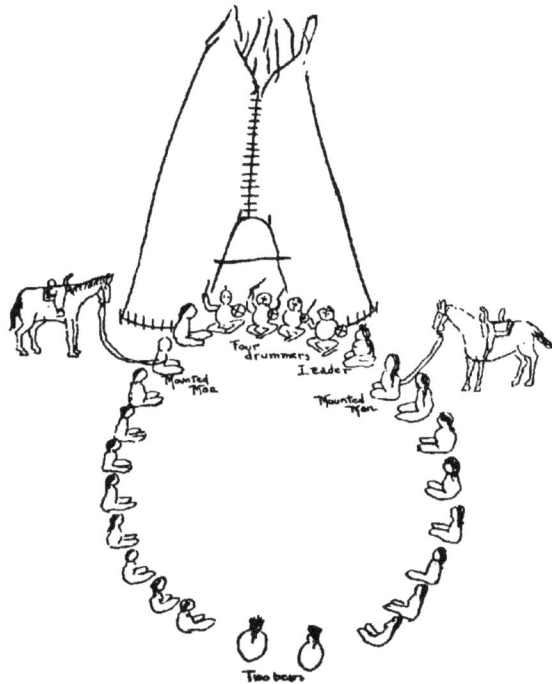

Source: Wissler, 1913

Sketch showing the formation of the all-brave-dogs before the tipi of a head man.

proceedings. The bundle in this new and modern format represents the goal of the process, and the ceremonialists guide the process. The bundle keepers are the hosts/hostesses of the process. They are regarded as stewards of the bundle/goal that is presented. The supporters who sit on the south and north side contribute to the process with their specific capabilities. As mentioned earlier, in a traditional ceremony, the women sit on the left side of the tipi and the men on the right side. In Blackfoot culture, women are regarded as representing the abstract and men the physical principles. This is reflected in the women's role of taking physical care of the bundle and the men's leading role of guiding the process.[3] In the "translated" form, this means that the supporters on the right side of the tipi contribute materially and financially to achieving the goal, and the supporters on the left side contribute the human resources.

The inner area of the floor plan contains the positions of the tobacco cutter, servers, and

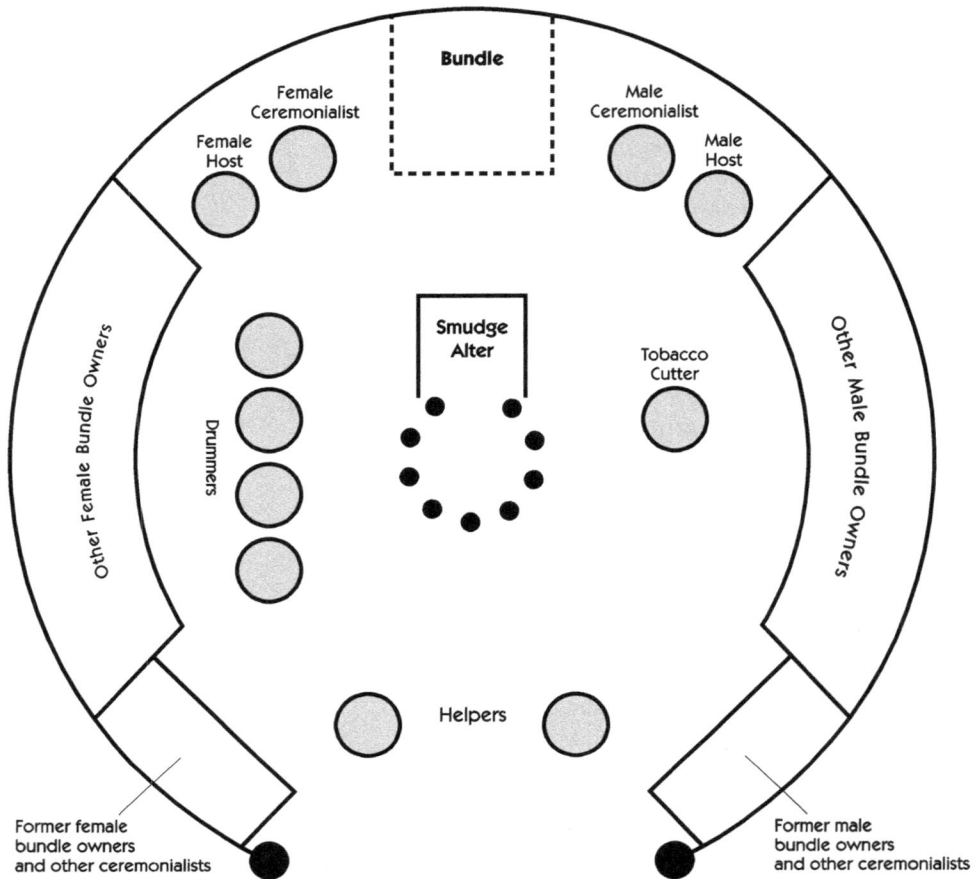

Traditional circle structure outline.

drummers. The tobacco cutter, as assistant to the ceremonialist, is, in the modern format, the person who keeps the records of the meeting and documents the agreements reached by all participants. Thus, the record keeper or assistant is central to the proper beginning and ending of the process. His or her helpers are equivalent to receptionists and others who help run a smooth organization. The positions of the drummers are filled by persons who represent supporting agencies or organizations. The advisory roles at the tipi doors are now taken by individuals who represent individuals in former positions in some way related to the goal.

This Blackfoot Circle Structure model thus gives all participants non-exclusive access to a process and ensures that they all contribute to the same goal. This means that all participants have to be clear about their roles in that process. Next to ensuring participation,[4] the model incorporates a specific quality of decision-making. It is based on a worldview that is not structured in a hierarchy and combines a balance of abstract and physical components that needs to be carefully maintained.[5] As pointed out in Chapter 4, in traditional ceremonies, this is demonstrated by the physical objects and materials held together in the bundle, as well as by the importance of following the proper protocol—the correct songs and paints in place. All together represent the physical and

Bundle Topic

Ceremonialist

Host

Ceremonialist

Host

Host Ceremonial Support

Host Ceremonial Support

Smudge Alter

Ceremonialist Technical Support

Ceremonialist Service Support

Advisors

Advisors

Service Technical Support

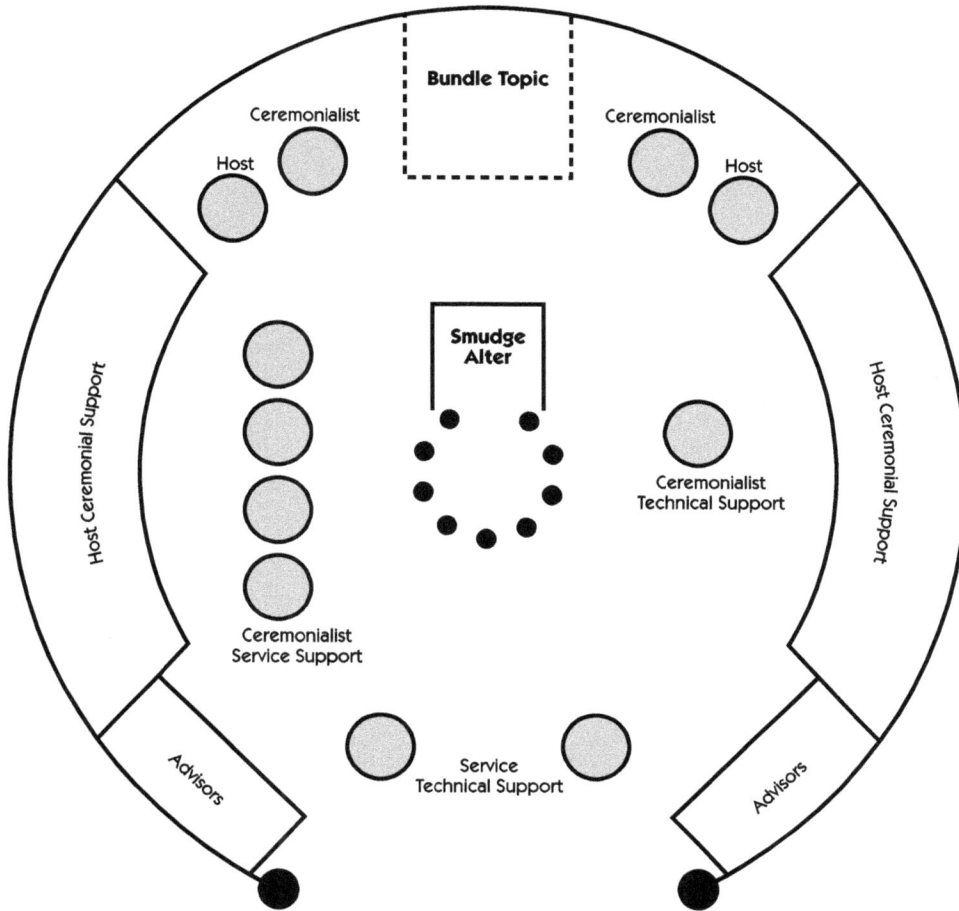

Modern circle structure outline.

abstract components, the animals and materials themselves, and the knowledge of them.[6] The traditional bundles were tools to deal with community issues, e.g., to solve conflicts or to help with solutions to certain concerns. Thus, they were central to the community's survival.

For this reason, the Blackfoot Circle Structure model allows for different possibilities than the management models presently applied in the Peigan community. It allows for participation by individuals willing to learn and take on the responsibilities that come with a specific position in the circle. The model is based on community participation because it allows for each individual's voice; it is not based on a hierarchical model, which favours experts and often outsiders to the community. Also, because of its traditional links to the survival of the community, the model assumes a certain authority that is still recognized by many Blackfoot people.

Thus, the Blackfoot Circle Structure model can be an optional management tool for all organizations striving to attain community-based goals. The model's central function is to find a solution to a specific concern, and its process is non-confrontational. Tipi etiquette rules are a modern-day manifestation of the model's rules of conduct.[7]

The Blackfoot Circle Structure model offers to Peigan Nation members and agencies an option for solving their concerns and achieve their goals.

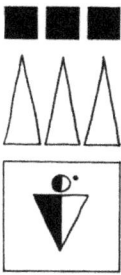

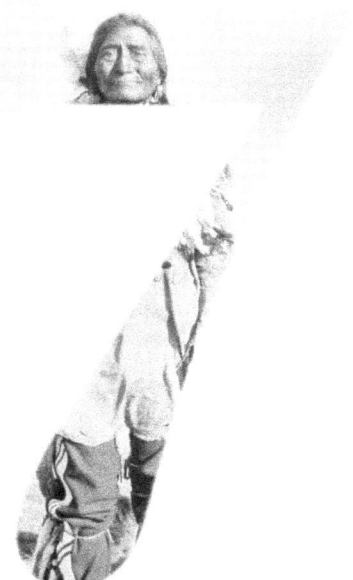

Healing, Health Services, and Health Providers

The previous chapters imply that, in traditional Blackfoot culture, health was defined in terms of survival. However, survival as an individual was only ensured in the collective, the extended family, the band, or the tribe. Survival was linked to the physical as well as to the abstract, and both were linked to all aspects of life, but especially in ceremonies. Individuals were taught to contribute to their group's survival and were rewarded for doing so, and Blackfoot people developed specific cultural traits accordingly. This chapter explores how disease, illness, and curing[1] were embedded in Blackfoot cultural structures. Furthermore, we will describe how Western culture, with different scientific and religious viewpoints on health and disease (including diagnosis, prognosis, and treatment), imposed on the Peigan people a new system of curing and illness prevention.

Traditional Blackfoot Medical Care

Many different ways of curing were used in traditional Blackfoot society, but three central categories of curative service delivery can be noted. The first involved knowledge of herbs and other natural remedies and was practised by skilled individuals who learned from a close relative and by their own trial and error. The second category involved services based on more practical, mechanical knowledge, like bone setting. The last category evolved around individuals and groups who went through a formalized training process that was closely linked to their roles as ceremonialists and holders of sacred bundles.

Some of these practices were historically documented by white observers[2] and by more recent Native informants. One of the first recorders in relation to all categories of medical intervention is Maximilian zu Wied, who comments on the Peigan/Blackfoot knowledge of herbal curing:

These Indians have some efficacious remedies derived from the vegetable kingdom, one of which is a whitish root from the Rocky Mountains, which is called, by the Canadians, rhubarb, which is said to resemble our rhubarb in its effect and taste, and likewise to act as an emetic. Another root is esteemed to be a powerful remedy against the bite of serpents. (1905, pp. 119–21)

At a much later date, certain elders give some indication of how much these traditional ways of herbal knowledge are still alive with the present-day Blackfoot people.[3] This information is confirmed by Hellson and Gadd (1974), who give an extensive taxonomy of plants used by the Blackfoot people, presented in six different categories: "1) plants in the religious ceremonial life, 2) plants in birth control, 3) plants in the treatment of sickness, 4) plants as horse medicine,

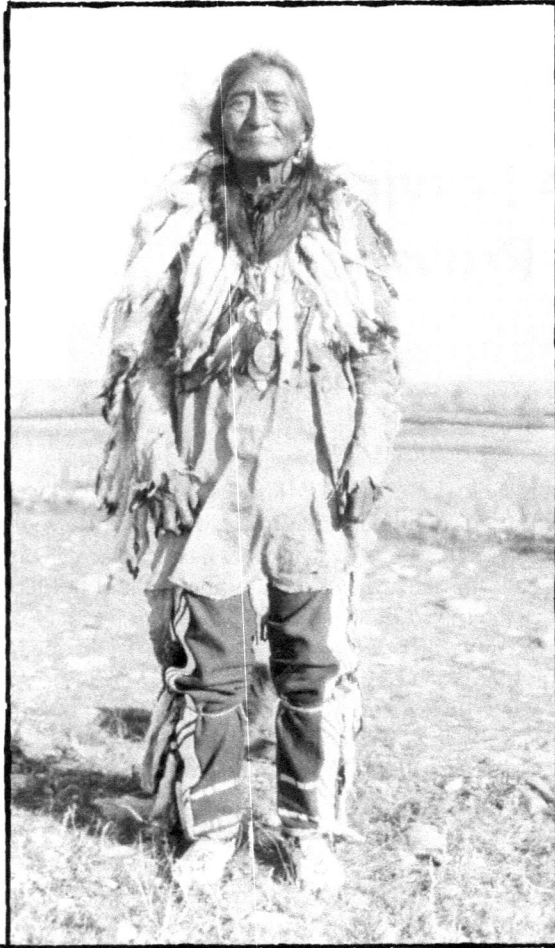

Courtesy of Provincial Archive of Manitoba, E. Morris Collection, 1907

"Brings Down the Sun" – Ceremonialist and Medicine Man of the North Peigan

5) plants in the diet, and 6) plants in folklore and craftways" (p. 2). The authors mention that some plants are used in more than one category. For example, the use of plant material to prevent conception and to assist in childbirth is widespread, although, in terms of the actual physical delivery, older women are the primary assistants.[4]

However, white men in first contact with the Blackfoot people showed greater interest in the more exotic appearances and activities of traditional curing experts, whom they called "medicine men."[5] Catlin describes a curing intervention in

1833 by a medicine man.[6] A similar observation is made by Maximilian zu Wied, who was present when a Peigan camp was attacked by Assiniboine and Cree in August 1833, just outside of Fort MacKenzie.[7] Considering these observers' limited knowledge and exposure to Blackfoot culture, it is obvious that traditional medical interventions cannot be regarded in the same way as curing based on the Western medical model.[8]

Additional information shows that medicine men were able to perform surgery, set bones, and administer appropriate medication, primarily based on their extensive herbal knowledge. However, the ability to apply these skills in a curative way was only one aspect of traditional Blackfoot medical interventions and was primarily applied to sudden, non-chronic afflictions that had a chance to be remedied fairly easily. Another approach to curing was used for conditions that were manifested by longer, unusual periods of suffering and for afflictions regarded as caused by a substance or something that could not be immediately explained. Most often, the first category of skills was combined with the second category of curing approaches.[9] For example, Denny observed a Blood Indian, shot through his shoulder blade, being cured by a medicine man who used both surgical skills and other elements:

> One Indian, a Blood, still living at the time of writing (1900), was shot right through the left lung, the bullet coming out below the shoulder-blade. He was attended by one of their own medicine men, as he could by no means be induced to let our police surgeon see him. This medicine man covered the wounded man with white mud from head to foot and spent a whole day drumming and singing over him, when he announced that he would bring the bad spirit out of the man in living shape. I then saw him inject from his mouth some substance into the bullet wound in the breast, and, withdrawing his hand from the wound, he held out a living white mouse. How he got it, I do not know. It was the first and only white mouse I ever saw in the country. However, the Indian finally recovered, and was still living a short time ago. (Denny (1944), p. 15)[10]

A man's ability to do this kind of surgery was closely connected with the power of an animal's spirit. This power could be directly applied by using a living animal, as in the previously mentioned case.[11] But, more often, the power was accessed by employing a symbolic representation of the animal, using particular body parts. Mentioned are skunk[12] and beaver skins,[13] owl feathers,[14] and eagle and grizzly bear claws. Eagle and bear claws were used for surgery, sometimes for retrieving bullets from wounds or to open abscesses; flints were used for incisions and amputations[15] during ceremonies and for puncturing.[16] Some of these materials were used like instruments for cutting, sewing, blowing, and puncturing. But they also had symbolic functions representing the specific curing powers of the animal spirit. Knowledge of how to set bones, particularly for arms and legs, was often handed down from father to son.[17]

Sometimes, these articles were not used singly but were combined with other things to produce a medicine bag or a kit.[18] For example, Jack Black Horse explains the function of the following pieces: a large and a small stone, a long bone tube, roots and tobacco, and a feather.[19]

Other reports show that the medicine man had the power to heal people who had been struck by lightning (Brasser 1974) or suffered from other ailments that were regarded as physical manifestations of taboo violations. In other instances, medicine men were thought to be able to foresee specific events. For example, Browne (1866) writes about meeting Rising Head (Ma-que-q-pas), a war chief of the Bloods who was a seer and could predict certain events.[20] Persons with such foresight and with the abilities to diagnose a problem with supernatural roots were most likely older, revered ceremonialists. As mentioned in Chapter 5, they would have participated in some form of transfer ceremony and would have acquired their curative abilities via the powers acquired in a vision or dream or obtained by payment. In these cases, curing was initiated by a combination of specific skills, but additionally through smudging, praying, singing of sacred songs, and the application of "real paint" (*assan* or red ochre) on the patient's body or face.[21]

Western Medical Services

One can assume, from the various descriptions of Blackfoot people, that, besides wounds inflicted by enemy weapons or accidental injuries (e.g., hunting or riding accidents), they were a relatively healthy population.[22] However, according to the wintercounts, there were also occasional periods of starvation and, at a later period, epidemics introduced by neighbouring tribes or by contact with infected trading goods. It was in this period, with the introduction of new diseases and changes of lifestyle (e.g., in living conditions, diet, and physical mobility) that the Blackfoot traditional health system started to falter.

At the same time, some curative services began to be provided by non-Natives, primarily fur traders and missionaries. Nevitt (1974), the first NWMP surgeon stationed in Fort Macleod, in 1874, rendered health services to some Blackfoot people.[23] However, at the same time, the Blackfoot people were still consulting their own health practitioners.[24] About ten years later, the condition of the Blackfoot people had changed drastically, and visitors found them in very poor condition

> … morally and spiritually, as well as physically. Physically, they were reduced to a state of practical starvation. The ration of beef and flour that the Government found it necessary to give them were not enough to keep from them the pangs of hunger…. The Hudson's Bay blanket had taken the place of the buffalo robe and the factory cotton flour sack had superseded the buckskin shirt and dress…. Little girls come to school with only one thin cotton garment on, beside the piece of blanket common to every Indian (Tims, in Stocken 1976, v–vi).

In addition to the general poverty caused by the vanishing of the buffalo and the peoples to restriction reserves, Natives were confronted by the introduction of unknown viruses, inadequate housing, and deficient diets, which led to the spread of new diseases like scrofula, tuberculosis, measles, and rheumatic fever.[25]

Thus, in the early contact period, interventions by Western-trained medical practitioners were sporadic and inadequate to the needs of the Native population they encountered.[26] Additionally, agents and missionaries used their influence to destroy existing traditional health structures. This was done by forbidding ceremonial activities, by undermining the role of traditional practitioners, and by simply destroying the whole social structure that supported the role of the medicine man; "Every effort was made by those who were in charge of Indians to discourage most of the methods used by the Medicine Man, but it took time to do this" (Graham 1991, p. 45).

In the summer of 1879, the first agency building was constructed on the North Peigan reserve by Indian agent Charles Kettles in order to give out rations for the Peigan. In August 1881, three Oblate missionaries arrived on the Peigan reserve and started building a cabin on the north side of the Oldman River (Doucet, no date). Missionaries sometimes took care of the sick, but their primary interest was not in curing, but in religious conversion and baptism before a sick person died. In June 1883, a Dr. Girard was appointed physician for the southern reserves by the Department of Indian Affairs, but it is not clear if he ever delivered services to the Peigan. It was the missionaries who kept the departmental medicine supplies for distribution when the doctor was absent.[27] A small hospital was built on the Blood reserve in 1893, but when Father Danis requested the same for the North Peigan reserve four years later, Indian Affairs refused. In 1898, a new doctor (Dr. Edwards), under the Indian agent Wilson, moved the medicine supplies from the Catholic mission to the band office. Three years later, he and another medical doctor (Dr. Lafferty) replaced the nuns and missionaries at the Blood hospital. In 1908, two other doctors set up office in Fort Macleod and Pincher Creek (Dr. Forbes and Dr. Turcotte), and the North Peigan were sometimes able to access their services. The first hospital on the North Peigan reserve was established in the house of the Anglican minister, near Victoria Home, the Anglican boarding school.[28] Peigan midwives were still active in the community and delivered babies until 1926, when the hospital was built.[29]

Canadian Government Health Bureaucracy

The Canadian government had accepted the transfer of responsibilities for "Indians and lands reserved for Indians" with the signing of the British North America Act in 1867. The government did not consider it their responsibility to include medical services for First Nations members.[30] It saw no legal obligation to provide for medicines, medical supplies, personnel, and hospitals, but rather felt a commitment on a humanitarian basis. This was manifested by ongoing changes in policies pertaining to medical care, and consequently its implementation was highly influenced by political and economic factors.

The first department of Indian Affairs was established in 1880, with Indian agents being its only employees on the local level. As mentioned above, these agents did not have the mandate to deal with medical care, lacked medical training, and had limited access to medical supplies. Occasionally, visiting doctors were available, but it was still the agent who used rations and visits to local physicians outside the reserve as control mechanisms. In 1904, the department appointed a general medical superintendent (Dr. Bryce), who in 1907 started an investigation into the conditions of residential schools. He considered most a breeding ground for tuberculosis and other infectious diseases, like measles, and suggested to the department closure of these institutions. However, missionary groups and Indian Affairs bureaucrats advancing their own agendas refused his suggestions, and not much changed. Dr. Bryce started the first nurse-visitor and health education programs for reserves in 1922. By that time, physicians in areas close to reserves were contracted on a fee-for-service basis to provide health care for Indians.

In 1927, the Medical Service Branch (MSB) under the Department of Indian Affairs was established with the mandate to structure health services for reserve residents. But it was still the

Indian agent on the local level who had the power to give permission if patients needed to be hospitalized or had to go to a sanatorium. By 1930, the first on-reserve nursing stations were established and MSB had grown to a bigger organization, with eleven medical officers and many contracted physicians. In 1936, the Department of Indian Affairs became part of the Department of Mines and Natural Resources, and in 1945 another restructuring move put Indian and Northern Health Services under the Department of National Health and Welfare. Any other affairs pertaining to First Nations stayed under the auspices of the Department of Indian Affairs and Northern Development (DIAND). Ten years later, MSB had a budget of $17 million. In 1962, the present-day structure was implemented and the Medical Services Branch delivered seven other programs outside of medical service delivery for First Nations members. A bureaucratic structure divided the country into regions and zones, and the North Peigan became part of the Alberta region, Southern Alberta zone—Treaty 7.

Since that time, registered Indians in Canada have received a range of free preventive and curative health services. Presently, the services are divided into insured and non-insured benefits, with the first covering hospital and physician care (including specialists) and the latter seven different programs. These include patient transportation (ambulance and taxi), prescription drugs, dental care, eyeglasses, prosthetic devices, medical appliances, and mental health services.

However, all these services (non-insured more so than insured benefits) are not secure, as they are regarded only as policies and can be changed on the basis of political decisions by the federal government.

Health Canada ①

Corporate Services Branch

Health Promotion and Programs Branch

Health Protection Branch

Medical Services Branch ②

First Nations and Inuit Health Programs Directorate

Program Policy, Transfer Secretariat & Planning Directorate

Health Policy and Information Directorate

Strategic Planning & Review Directorate

Manage-ment Services Directorate

Non-insured Health Benefits Directorate

International Affairs Directorate

Communications Directorate

Inter-governmental Affairs Directorate

Occupational & Environmental Health Services Directorate

Health Advisory Services Directorate

Women's Health Bureau

Regional Offices

Zones

On-Reserve Health Centres, Health Administration

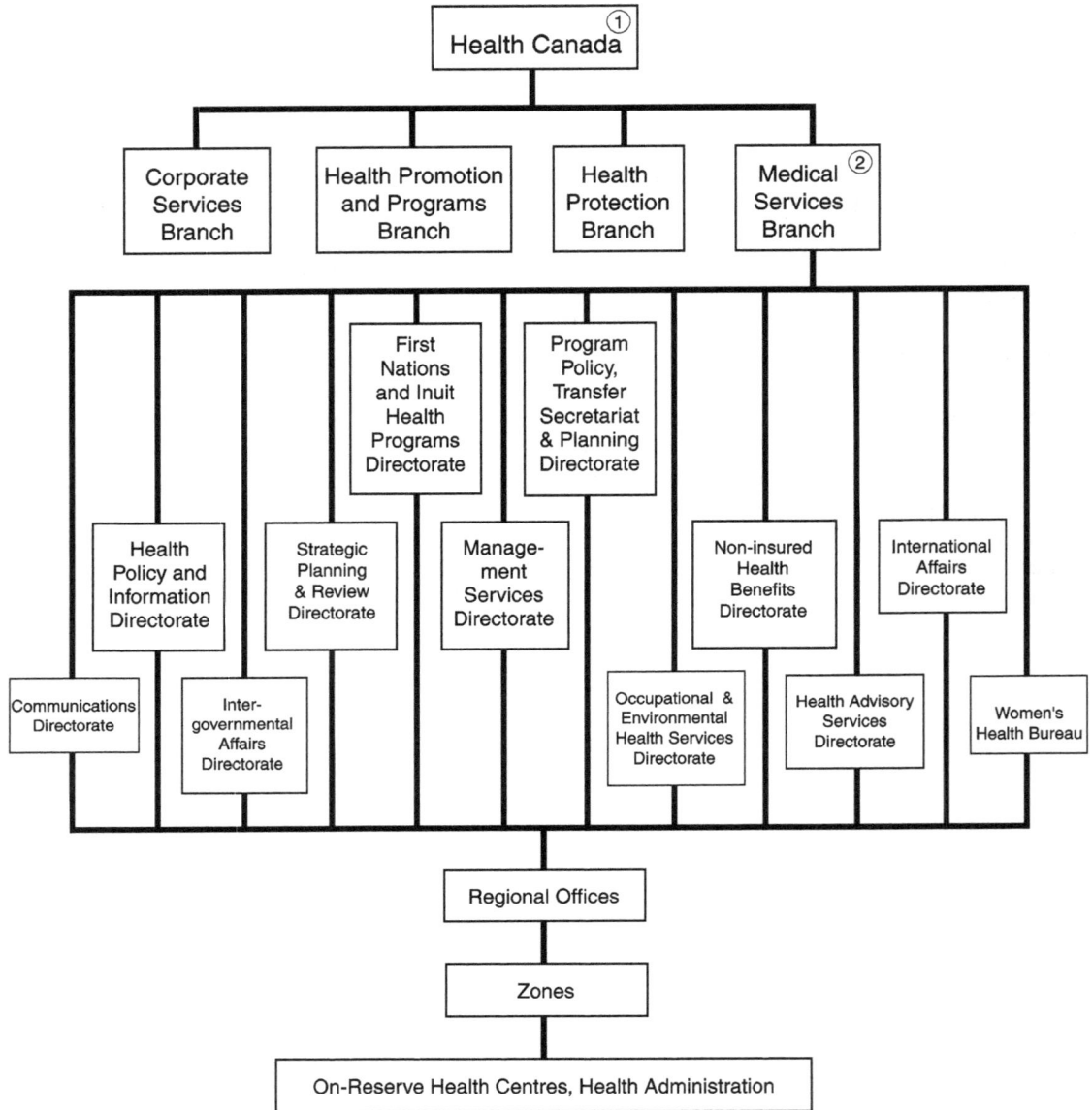

① Previously Department of National Health and Welfare

② MSB clients are the Inuit and status Indians, all residents of the Yukon, federal public servants, international travellers, civil aviation personnel, and disaster victims.

Medical Services Branch structure.

Credit Rob Storeshaw

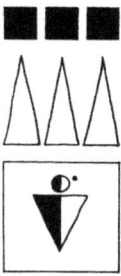

The Blackfoot Circle Structure Model and its Application to Health Administration

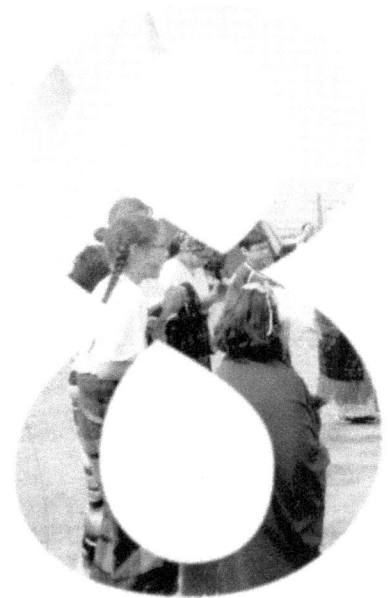

As pointed out in previous chapters, the existing administrative structures for delivery of health services to the Peigan people are based on a historical model that was alien to and imposed on the community. Additionally, this administrative structure does not include grassroots community participation. Its hierarchical structure allows input by "health experts" only, who are either the practitioners working on a local level in the health posts or administrators working locally or at the zone level. Even though some of these individuals are Native and may still have a strong connection to their community, they have to operate within a system that has extremely limited community input. Thus, the services developed out of this Western-based structure with its Western values are not connected to the traditional values of those they are trying to serve. Rather, the services may be misunderstood, misused, not respected and, finally, not accessed.[1]

We argue that the Blackfoot Circle Structure is the more appropriate model to use in structuring health services for the Peigan people.[2] The following paragraphs define this model and outline how it can be applied as an administrative tool for future Peigan health services.

The bundle/goal for this circle structure is defined as health services for the Peigan community. The aim is for all participants invited into the circle to be responsible for their contribution in achieving this goal. This research suggests one standard format that allows for certain individuals to take their place inside the circle.[3]

The role of the ceremonialist and host will be the same through all circle meetings. The ceremonialist on the right side, who was traditionally responsible for guiding the decision-making process, is the chairperson of the health board. He or she is in charge of keeping the protocol in place and ensuring that all bylaws of the organization are followed. His or her assistant (the traditional role of the tobacco cutter) is the secretary of the board, who records the proceedings and all agreements made by the participants (e.g., resolutions). The assistant's helpers are other employees of the health board, for example, the secretary and other administrative assistants. The host, who is the caretaker of the bundle on a daily basis, is the administrator or executive director of health administration. He or she, with the help of the assistants, informs the participants about the meetings and makes sure that each participant has received enough training to understand his or her role in the process and that they sit in the right positions. On the other side of the bundle/goal (which symbolizes the abstract elements of the circle), the vice-chairperson takes his or her seat. The role of the vice-chairperson focuses on the importance of the mandate of the organization, with the persons taking the position on his or her side being one or both researchers,[4] as they were involved in the development of the model. Once a person is trained in the model, he or she can take over the responsibility and ensure that the guidelines of the model are followed.

On the right-hand side of the circle sit all the individuals who contribute to the topic in

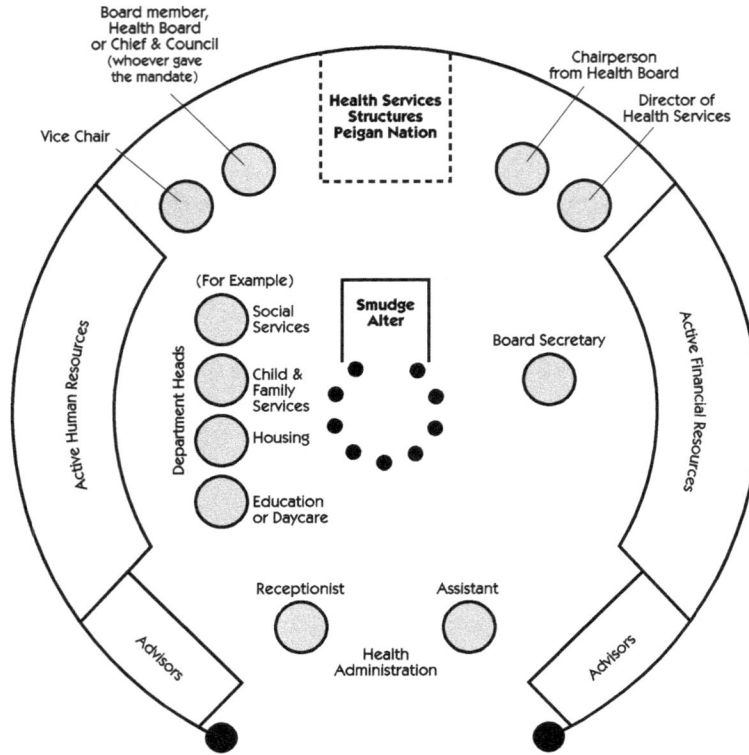

Health services circle structure outline.

material or financial ways. On the opposite side will be seated individuals who contribute their knowledge of the topic. These guests can be from inside or outside the community and can be personally involved or represent certain agencies or organizations. They take an active role in achieving the goals of the Peigan health board and administration, which is different from the role of advisor. The latter are possible former board members, or retired professionals who take on an advisory role. They have a veto right to interrupt or influence the outcome of the procedure, but commonly function in the role of observers.

The traditional role of the drummers is then taken by individuals who represent various agencies on the reserve. Again, who is invited to take these positions will depend on the specific topic to be discussed. These participants can represent off-reserve organizations, and their main role is to help the chairperson find a way to implement some of the objectives reached in discussion by all participants in the circle.

The meeting starts with a short announcement by the host (administrator or chief executive) to explain the purpose of the circle. The chairperson of the board (ceremonialist) lays out the rules for the proceedings, the roles of each participant, and the need to focus on the goal of the meeting. The chairperson starts the meeting with a symbolic act; depending on the topic discussed and the comfort level of the participants, this could be a smudge.[5] The chairperson also indicates when the meeting has ended, when all participants have reached a consensus. This could be symbolized by the consensus being recorded in the minutes or by signing with a seal, comparable to smoking a pipe at the end of a traditional ceremony. This would mean that all agreements made in the circle structure are binding for all participants.

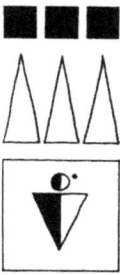

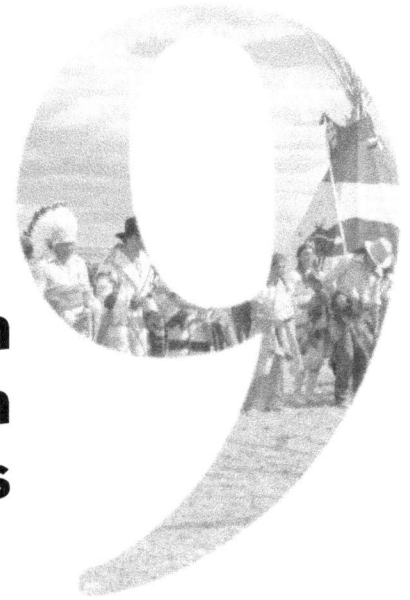

An Application to Mediation Processes in Child Protection and in Business Practices

The first application of the model presented is currently used by Calgary Rockyview Child and Family Services in dispute cases related to child protection and guardianship issues.

In this application, the Child Welfare Act is the central topic in place of the traditional bundle that symbolizes the guiding principle for the mediation process. On the right hand side of the circle, the position of the ceremonialist is taken by a person who has the transferred rights to facilitate the mediation and the formal permission to do so. Next to him or her sits the host, who is the parent or guardian applying for the child's permanent guardianship. On the left side, the position of the ceremonialist is presented by a person who carries the mandate for the agency and who has to uphold the law. This might be the director of Child and Family Services or someone who is in a similar position and a department head. On his or her right side, the co-host is placed. This role is taken by the social worker involved in the case.

Back to the right side of the circle, sitting next to the host, family members and friends who are supporting the guardianship application of the applicant, take their seat. On the opposite side, various professionals who are resources to the social worker will be placed. At the entrance to the circle, advisors will be seated. These are individuals who have gone previously through the process of guardianship, have been foster parents, and who have formerly worked in the area of child protection. These individuals take on the

role of the former ceremonialist or elder ceremonialist in the traditional circle structure model.

The traditional role of the drummers is occupied by representatives of various agencies who are involved in the specific case under review. These might be social workers involved with the family, a psychologist who has worked with the child, an elder who has supported the family, or a teacher. The representatives should be involved with the case—be it the parents or guardian or the child—but they should be working with agencies other than the Child and Family Services that is setting up this mediation process. The helpers in this case will be representatives of the Child and Family Services agency and will assist the ceremonialist in running a successful mediation process. The individual who will take minutes for the meeting sits in the position of the tobacco cutter in the traditional circle structure ceremony.

Figure 9 shows the outline of this culturally appropriate mediation process. It has been in use since 1999 and has been practised in more than ten cases, particularly, when guardianship of a Native child under the jurisdiction of Calgary Rockyview Child and Family Services has been under dispute.

Figure 10 shows the traditional circle structure model applied to present-day business practices, particularly for mediation processes. Here, the bundle is reflected by the mission statement or statement of intent of the organization that requires a mediation process. Again, in this

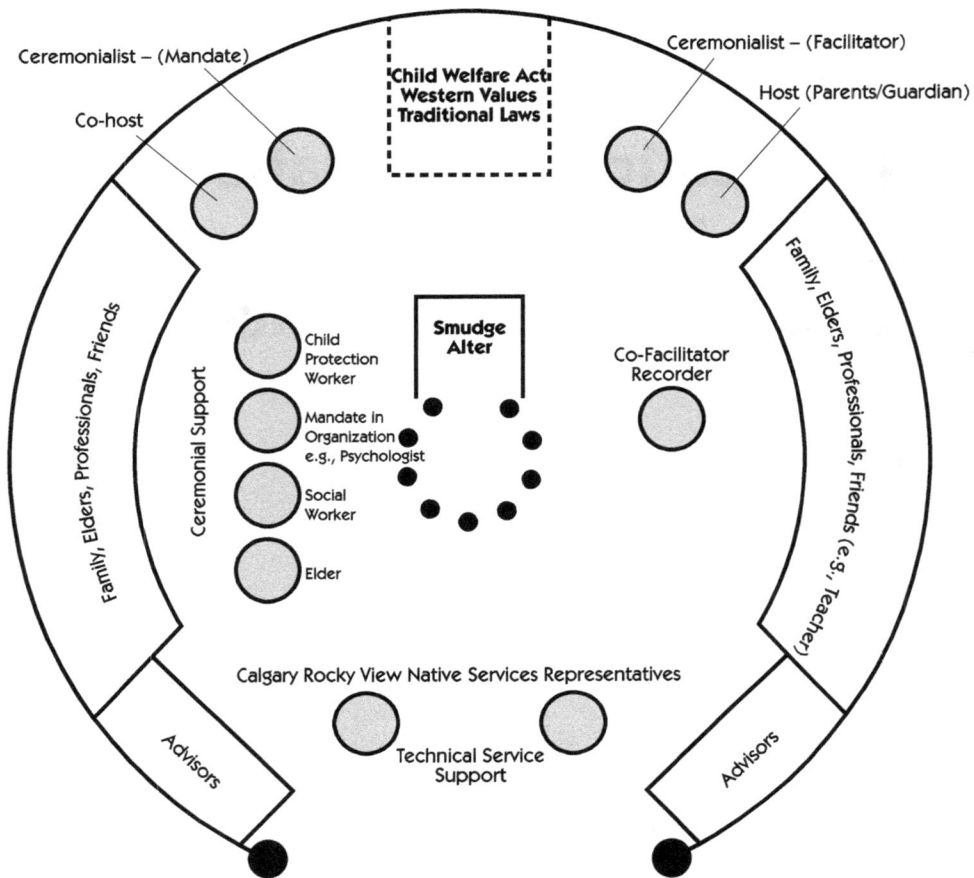

Child Welfare circle structure outline.

application, certain individuals have particular roles to take on. On the right side of the bundle, the executive officer, the person who is chiefly responsible for the practical application of the by-laws of the organization, takes a seat. Next to this position sits another member of the organization or a leading staff person. Opposite these two positions, on the left half of the circle, the chairperson of the organization takes a seat. This could be the chair of the board, the president, or anyone else who holds up the mandate of the organization. Next to him or her sits again a staff person, primarily someone who works with policy and staff development issues.

The positions that are in the traditional circle on both sides occupied by the male and female bundle owners are in this case taken by share-holders or staff of the organization. The seats at the entrance of the circle, in opposition to the bundle, are reserved for former executives of the organization. They embody the roles of elders in the traditional structure and are advisors in this mediation process.

In the middle of the circle, the role of the tobacco cutter is taken on by the secretary of the organization. The positions of the helpers and drummers are taken by administrative personnel and various department chairs, respectively.

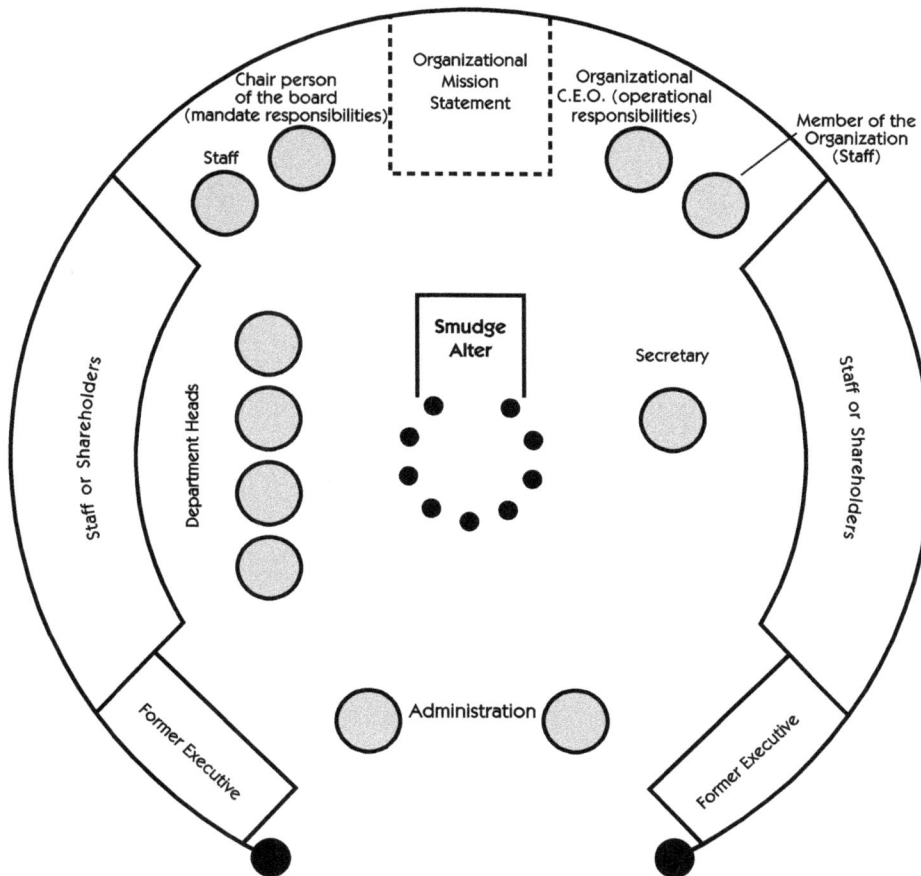

Business practices circle structure outline.

To date, this application has been presented to several business organizations in the energy sector and the oil and gas industry who wish to negotiate business deals with various Native communities and try to implement more cultural appropriate mediation processes.

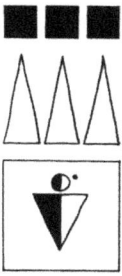

Conclusion

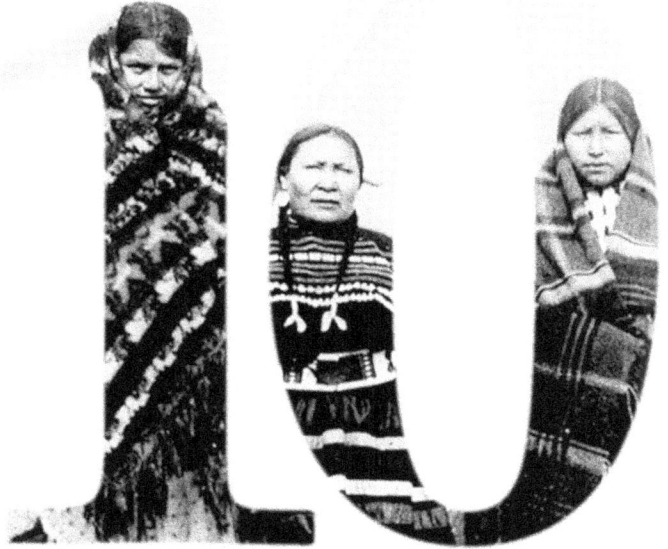

his model developed from the analysis of the history and social structure of past days of the Peigan/Blackfoot culture and its present-day, still practised, ceremonies. Aside from their spiritual importance, these ceremonies were always intended to find common solutions, to elicit agreements, and to establish a common understanding for future actions of the community. In this sense, they presented condensed information of Peigan/Blackfoot indigenous knowledge.

Based on this information, several applications of this model for mediation and conflict-resolution situations are presented. They are presently practised in dispute cases in child protection, in business negotiations in some industries and in sentencing circles in the justice system. They are particularly used in situations when Native and non-Native worlds are coming together and cultural translation becomes a central issue for mutual understanding. We feel that this model has value beyond bridging the gap between these two worlds and suggest that it offers an option for future directions by establishing culturally appropriate procedures toward Native self-government.

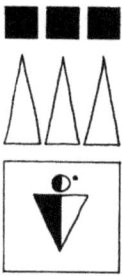

Appendices

Appendix A: Creation Story

The stories I heard were from my dad and my grandmother. And I heard some of these stories from Mike Swims Under and other people that came to visit our house when we were young. And they talked about Napi, and some of the Napi stories that I hear and how they relate to today. And part of the story goes:

"At the beginning of time, people and Creation on the world, met with and interacted with the Star People, the stars, the moon, and the different planets. They all used to interact and live together. But at one point the kids from the earth played a little too rough. What they did was they killed one of the star children. So the people from the above got mad and they moved away. They split the earth and the heavens. They did not want to interact with the people on earth. When they split up they told Creator to punish the people on the world by flooding the world. So it started raining. It rained for a long time. Water started collecting in different places, and got deeper. And Napi and his friends, the animals, they started looking for high ground. And it got to a point where Napi was caught on top of a mountain, on the rock, and he took his rope and he roped the clouds and he stopped the rain. And that rope was the rainbow.

And then he asked the animals to go down and get some mud for him. The duck flew way up in the air, and he dived into the water. He came back up and he didn't have any mud in his hand. He asked other animals. Eventually he asked the muskrat and the muskrat went down. All of a sudden the muskrat came out on his back gasping for air. They pulled him ashore, and when they looked in his paw, sure enough there was some mud. And anyway Creator gave him a present; he gave him hands like humans.

But at the same time he used that mud to recede the waters down. And as the waters receded, life got going on earth again. And as life got going, you find that Napi put us Piikani out in the prairie. And you find these mushrooms; they are called puff balls. They are a round sort of mushroom that are out in the prairie. All these things that you find like that, make the old people say: 'We're a part of that Star child that was killed and were left on earth, so that we remember what happened.'

That's why the fungus is part of Piikani bundles, to remind us.

From Crowshoe (1997c)

Appendix B: First Contacts Between White Men and Blackfoot

1690–91   A Hudson's Bay fur trader named Henry Kelsey (1670–1724) possibly met the Blackfoot on the Alberta/Saskatchewan border. He called them Naywatames. The Hudson's Bay Company later used the term Archithinues for the Blackfoot. At that time, the Blackfoot suffered from defeat in war with other tribes because they lacked guns.

1731–41   Sieur de la Verendrye, a Northwest Fur Company agent and explorer, went as far as the forks of the Saskatchewan River and crossed the Great Plains to the Missouri. He might have met Blackfoot.

1750?   Another Northwest Fur Company trader, Alexander Henry, possibly had contact with the Peigans.

1754–55   A Hudson's Bay Company fur trader named Anthony Henday (Hendry) is recorded as the first white man to meet the Blackfoot. He spent the winter in western Alberta with the intention of convincing the Blackfoot to trade with the Hudson's Bay Company. He visited, at present-day Red Deer, a Blood camp with 322 lodges. The Blackfoot, however, were not interested in trading. They had horses, and the buffalo were plentiful.

1772–73   Matthew Cocking, a Hudson's Bay Company fur trader, spent the winter with the Blackfoot Confederacy. He found them to be friendly and hospitable. Like Henday, Cocking failed to convince the Blackfoot to trade.

1779   William Tomison, met a Peigan chief at Buckingham House, which is now Dewberry, Alberta.

1792–93   Peter Fidler, a Hudson's Bay explorer and surveyor, met Blood Indians at the Red Deer River. He lived with the Peigan. A Hudson's Bay trading post was established at Chesterfield House, which is now Empress, Alberta. The Blackfoot went there to trade pemmican for guns. In 1801–02, Fidler met the Pekanow or Muddy Water Indians (possibly Peigans) for the first time at Rocky Mountain House.

1795–1806   Lewis and Clarke were American explorers who met the Blackfeet in present-day Montana. The explorers shot and killed a Blackfoot, which lead to the persecution of all white people for twenty-five years.

1807–10   An explorer and map-maker, David Thompson, met a Cree named Saukamappee, who lived with the Peigan and tells how the Peigan saw their first horse around 1730. Thompson also met a Peigan chief in Rocky Mountain House, named Kootenae Appe.

1831   James Kipp, an American Fur Company trader, built Fort Peigan at the mouth of the Marias River. He married a Mandan woman, named Earth Woman. His son, Joseph Kipp, became a trader at Fort Whoop-Up.

1833–34   Maximilian, Prince zu Wied, and his painter Karl Bodmer met Blackfoot, Blood, and Peigan tribe members at Fort McKenzie. They are the first to publish detailed descriptions and images of aspects of Blackfoot culture.

1833–42   Alexander Culbertson, another American Fur Company trader, was chief manager at Fort McKenzie. He married a woman from the Blood tribe named Medicine Snake Woman, Natamista Iksana. In 1846, Culbertson built Fort Benton.

1839–47   A Wesleyan missionary named Robert T. Rundle was stationed between Edmonton and Banff. He worked primarily with the Stonies, but did have contact with the Blackfoot.

1840–57   John Palliser, an explorer, made two trips into Blackfoot territory, where he possibly met the Peigan. On his second trip, he was the leader of a British government expedition and was accompanied by James Hector, M.D.

1845   Father de Smet met the Blackfoot.

1846–48   At Fort Edmonton, the artist Paul Kane met the Blackfoot, "Pay-guns," and the Bloods. Kane also met the trader Jimmy Jock Bird at Rocky Mountain Fort.

1859   The Earl of Southesk, James Carnegie, an explorer and adventurer, met the Blackfoot at Fort Edmonton.

1863–75   Constantine-Michael Scollen (O.M.I.) was in the Macleod and High River area. He built a mission in Calgary in 1873. Scollen was present at the signing of Treaty 7. He was originally an Oblate father but left the order in 1885.

1865–69   Father Lacombe (O.M.I.) arrived in Edmonton in 1852. He worked with the Blackfoot people and reported on the smallpox epidemic that came from Fort Benton and killed nearly half of the Blackfoot Confederacy (3,500 people). He also reported on the scarlet fever plague, which claimed the lives of more than a thousand Blackfoot.

1869   J.J. Healy was a whisky trader, freight sheriff, newspaper publisher, ferryman, and prospector and built Fort Whoop-Up.

1870s   John McDougall, a Wesleyan missionary, was also present at the signing of Treaty 7.

1874   Richard B. Nevitt, an NWMP surgeon, was posted for four years in Fort Macleod. He treated police members, settlers, and Blackfoot people.

1874–85   Sir Cecil E. Denny came to Fort Macleod with the NWMP and later became an Indian agent. He describes the signing of Treaty 7 and notes that the Blackfoot nation numbered 8,000. In April 1885, he resigned as Indian agent.

1877–   Jimmy Jock Bird (1832–1891), a half-breed Cree, interpreted at the signing of Treaty 7 at Blackfoot Crossing. He was a Hudson's Bay Company trader around Fort Union. He translated for Robert T. Rundle and Pierre de Smet, who were missionaries. Bird lived on the Peigan reserve and was married to a Cree woman.

1877   W.F. Butler, a NWMP member, estimated 4,000 people in the Blackfoot Confederacy.

1878–1910   Leon Doucet (O.M.I.) lived with the Peigan and Blackfoot and wrote a notebook on Blackfoot people, vocabulary, and grammar.

1879   Edgar Dewdney, an Indian commissioner, visited Blackfoot Crossing and found the Natives to be suffering terribly; "after eating all their dogs, [they] were reduced to eating gophers and mice."

1889   S.F. Fraser, M.D., was a NWMP assistant surgeon at Fort Macleod.

1916–27   Jean-Louis Levern (O.M.I.) lived among the Peigan and wrote dictionaries and grammar books in Blackfoot. He also produced writings on the Blackfoot people.

Appendix C: Legend of Star Boy (Later, Poia, Scarface)

We know not when the Sun-dance had its origin. It was long ago, when the Blackfeet used dogs for beasts of burden instead of horses; when they stretched the legs and bodies of their dogs on sticks to make them large, and when they used stones instead of wooden pegs to hold down their lodges. In those days, during the moon of flowers (early summer), our people were camped near the mountains. It was a cloudless night and a warm wind blew over the prairie. Two young girls were sleeping in the long grass outside the lodge. Before daybreak, the eldest sister, So-at-sa-ki (Feather Woman), awoke. The Morning Star was just rising from the prairie. He was very beautiful, shining through the clear air of early morning. She lay gazing at this wonderful star, until he seemed very close to her, and she imagined that he was her lover. Finally she awoke her sister, exclaiming, "Look at the Morning Star! He is beautiful and must be very wise. Many of the young men have wanted to marry me, but I love only the Morning Star." When the leaves were turning yellow (autumn), So-at-sa-ki became very unhappy, finding herself with child. She was a pure maiden, although not knowing the father of her child. When the people discovered her secret, they taunted and ridiculed her until she wanted to die. One day while the geese were flying southward, So-at-sa-ki went alone to the river for water. As she was returning home, she beheld a young man standing before her in the trail. She modestly turned aside to pass, but he put forth his hand, as if to detain her, and she said angrily, "Stand aside! None of the young men have ever before dared to stop me." He replied, "I am the Morning Star. One night, during the moon of flowers, I beheld you sleeping in the open and loved you. I have now come to ask you to return with me to the sky, to the lodge of my father, the Sun, where we will live together, and you will have no more trouble."

Then So-at-sa-ki remembered the night in spring, when she slept outside the lodge, and now realised that Morning Star was her husband. She saw in his hair a yellow plume, and in his hand a juniper branch with a spider web hanging from one end. He was tall and straight and his hair was long and shining. His beautiful clothes were of soft-tanned skins, and from them came a fragrance of pine and sweet grass. So-at-sa-ki replied hesitatingly, "I must first say farewell to my father and mother." But Morning Star allowed her to speak to no one. Fastening the feather in her hair and giving her the juniper branch to hold, he directed her to shut her eyes. She held the upper strand of the spider web in her hand and placed her feet upon the lower one. When he told her to open her eyes, she was in the sky. They were standing together before a large lodge. Morning Star said, "This is the home of my father and mother, the Sun and the Moon," and bade her enter. It was day-time and the Sun was away on his long journey, but the Moon was at home. Morning Star addressed his mother saying, "One night I beheld this girl sleeping on the prairie. I loved her and she is now my wife." The Moon welcomed So-at-sa-ki to their home. In the evening, when the Sun Chief came home, he also gladly received her. The Moon clothed So-at-so-ki in a soft-tanned buckskin dress, trimmed with elk-teeth . She also presented her with wristlets of elk-teeth and an elk-skin robe, decorated with the sacred paint, saying, "I give you these because you have married our son." So-at-sa-ki lived happily in the sky with Morning Star, and learned many wonderful things. When her child was born, they called him Star Boy. The Moon then gave So-at-sa-ki a root digger, saying, "This should be used only by pure women. You can dig all kinds of roots with it, but I warn you not to dig up the large turnip growing near the home of the Spider Man. You have now a child, and it would bring unhappiness to us all."

Everywhere So-at-sa-ki went, she carried her baby and the root digger. She often saw the large turnip, but was afraid to touch it. One day, while passing the wonderful turnip, she thought of the mysterious warning of the Moon, and became curious to see what might be underneath. Laying her baby on the ground, she dug until her root digger stuck fast. Two large cranes came flying from the east. So-at-sa-ki besought them to help her. Thrice she called in vain, but upon the fourth call, they circled and lighted beside her. The chief crane sat upon one side of the turnip and his wife on the other. He took hold of the turnip with his long sharp bill, and moved it backwards and forwards, singing the medicine song, "This root is sacred. Whenever I dig, my roots are sacred."

He repeated this song to the north, south, east and west. After the fourth song, he pulled up the turnip. So-at-sa-ki looked through the hole and beheld the earth. Although she had not known it, the turnip had filled the same hole, through which Morning Star had brought her into the sky. Looking down, she saw the camp of the Blackfeet, where she had lived. She sat for a long while gazing at the old familiar scenes. The young men were playing games. The women were tanning hides and making lodges, gathering berries on the hills, and crossing the meadows to the river for water. When she turned to go home, she was crying, for she felt lonely and longed to be back again upon the green prairies with her own people. When So-at-sa-ki arrived at the lodge, Morning Star and his mother were waiting. As soon as Morning Star looked at his wife, he exclaimed, "You have dug up the sacred turnip!" When she did not reply, the Moon said, "I warned you not to dig up the turnip, because I love Star Boy and do not wish to part with him." Nothing more was said, because it was day-time and the great Sun Chief was still away on his long journey. In the evening, when he entered the lodge, he exclaimed, "What is the matter with my daughter? She looks sad and must be in trouble." So-at-sa-ki replied, "Yes, I am homesick, because I have to-day looked down upon my people." Then the Sun Chief was angry and said to Morning Star, "If she has disobeyed, you must send her home." The Moon interceded for So-at-sa-ki, but the Sun answered, "She can no longer be happy with us. It is better for her to return to her own people." Morning Star led So-at-sa-ki to the home of the Spider Man, whose web had drawn her up to the sky. He placed on her head the sacred Medicine Bonnet, which is worn only by pure women. He laid Star Boy on her breast, and wrapping them both in the elk-skin robe, bade her farewell, saying, "We will let you down into the centre of the Indian camp and the people will behold you as you come from the sky." The Spider Man then carefully let them down through the hole to the earth.

It was an evening in midsummer, during the moon when the berries are ripe, when So-at-sa-ki was let down from the sky. Many of the people were outside their lodges, when suddenly they beheld a bright light in the northern sky. They saw it pass across the heavens and watched, until it sank to the ground. When the Indians reached the place, where the star had fallen, they saw a strange looking bundle. When the elk-skin cover was opened, they found a woman and her child. So-at-sa-ki was recognised by her parents. She returned to their lodge and lived with them, but never was happy. She used to go with Star Boy to the summit of a high ridge, where she sat and mourned for her husband. One night she remained alone upon the ridge. Before day-break, when Morning Star arose from the plains, she begged him to take her back. Then he spoke to her, "You disobeyed and therefore cannot return to the sky. Your sin is the cause of your sorrow and has brought trouble to you and your people."

Before So-at-sa-ki died, she told all these things to her father and mother, just as I now tell them to you. Star Boy's grandparents also died. Although born in the home of the Sun, he was very poor. He had no clothes, not even moccasins to wear. He was so timid and shy that he never played with other children. When the Blackfeet moved camp, he always followed barefoot, far behind the rest of the tribe. He feared to travel with the other people, because the other boys stoned and abused him. On his face was a mysterious scar, which became more marked as he grew older. He was ridiculed by everyone and in derision was called Poia (Scarface).

When Poia became a young man, he loved a maiden of his own tribe. She was very beautiful and the daughter of a leading chief. Many of the young men wanted to marry her, but she refused them all. Poia sent this maiden a present, with the message that he wanted to marry her, but she was proud and disdained his love. She scornfully told him, she would not accept him as her lover, until he would remove the scar from his face. Scarface was deeply grieved by the reply. He consulted with an old medicine woman, his only friend. She revealed to him, that the scar had been placed on his face by the Sun God, and that only the Sun himself could remove it. Poia resolved to go to the home of the Sun God. The medicine woman made moccasins for him and gave him a supply of pemmican.

"Poia journeyed alone across the plains and through the mountains, enduring many hardships and great dangers. Finally he came to the Big Water (Pacific Ocean). For three days and three nights he lay upon the shore, fasting and praying to the Sun God. On the evening of the fourth day, he beheld a bright trail leading across the water. He travelled this path until he drew near the home of the Sun, when he hid himself and waited. In the morning, the great Sun Chief came from his lodge, ready for his daily journey. He did not recognise Poia. Angered at beholding a creature from the earth, he said to the Moon, his wife, "I will kill him, for he comes from a good-for-nothing-race, but she interceded and saved his life. Morning Star, their only son, a young man with a handsome face and beautifully dressed, came forth from the lodge. He brought with him dried sweet grass, which he burned as incense. He first placed Poia in the sacred smoke, and then led him into the presence of his father and mother, the Sun and the Moon. Poia related the story of his long journey, because of his rejection by the girl he loved. Morning Star then saw how sad and worn he looked. He felt sorry for him and promised to help him.

Poia lived in the lodge of the Sun and Moon with Morning Star. Once, when they were hunting together, Poia killed seven enormous birds, which had threatened the life of Morning Star. He presented four of the dead birds to the Sun and three to the Moon. The Sun rejoiced, when he knew that the dangerous birds were killed, and the Moon felt so grateful, that she besought her husband to repay him. On the intercession of Morning Star, the Sun God consented to remove the scar. He also appointed Poia as his messenger to the Blackfeet, promising if they would give a festival (Sun-dance) in his honour, once every year, he would restore their sick to health. He taught Poia the secrets of the Sun-dance, and instructed him in the prayers and songs to be used. He gave him two raven feathers to wear as a sign that he came from the Sun, and a robe of soft-tanned elk-skin, with the warning that it must be worn only by a virtuous woman. She can then give the Sun-dance and the sick will recover. Morning Star gave him a magic flute and a wonderful song, with which he would be able to charm the heart of the girl he loved.

Poia returned to the earth and the Blackfeet camp by the Wolf Trail (Milky Way), the short path to the earth. When he had fully instructed his people concerning the Sun-dance, the Sun God took him back to the sky with the girl he loved. When Poia returned to the home of the Sun, the Sun God made him bright and beautiful, just like his father, Morning Star. In those days Morning Star and his son could be seen together in the east. Because Poia appears first in the sky, the Blackfeet often mistake him for his father, and he is therefore sometimes called Poks-o-piks-o-aks, Mistake Morning Star.

From McClintock (1968), pp. 491–99

Appendix D: The Elk-Woman

Blood Version

This medicine-bonnet was given to a woman who was camping near the Mountains. One day while her husband was away she heard an Elk whistling in the woods. At another time when her husband was away, a man came to the lodge and asked her to go away with him. He told her that he was the Elk that she had heard, and that, if she would go away with him, he would give her some medicine. To this promise she finally consented and went with him into the brush, where he explained to her the whole ceremony. He told her all about the medicine-bonnet, calling in many animals to help give the woman some power. Among these was the Crane, who offered the use of his bill to dig the medicine-turnip. He said his bill was to be carried on the back like the bunch of feathers on his own neck. Then the Crane proceeded to dig with his bill, and as he did so he sang a song, "I wish to be on level ground."

A robe made of elk-skin, used by the woman in the ceremony, is to represent the Elk himself. The bunches of feathers placed around the bonnet are to represent the prongs of the horns. There are about six bunches in all. In front is hung a doll with quill-work upon it. A white-rock arrowpoint and some ear-rings are hung on the side. There are also two little dolls tied on near the feathers. Weasel-tails hang down by the side. Feathers of the owl are used in making up the bunches on the side of the bonnet, while behind is hung the skin of a woodpecker (?) and part of the tail of a wild-cat. There should also be part of the tail of a white buffalo tied on somewhere.

All of these parts were contributed by the animals called together by the man who took the woman into the brush, and each of these animals sang a song as they gave them. The buffalo was there also, and gave its hoofs, which were tied to the end of the digging-stick.

You will see all these things upon the medicine-bonnet; but the present one used by the Blood Indians is a little different from that used by the Peigan.

Peigan Version

You are asking me about the badger and the medicine-bonnet? Well, the badger-skin is used as a case in which to put the bonnet, but the badger-skin is a new addition to this. It was dreamed not so very long ago. This badger-skin should always be painted red, and it is necessary to go through a ceremony when it is painted. But now I must tell you about the bonnet.

There was once an Elk who was deserted by his wife. When he found that she was gone, he went out to look for her, and finally saw her in the thick woods. He was very angry and wished to kill her: so he walked toward her singing a song. Now this was a medicine-song, and he intended that its power should kill his wife. He had great power. The ground was very hard; but at every step his feet sank deeper into it. Now his wife was frightened; but she had some power also. She began to sing a song, and as she did so she turned into a woman. In her new form she wore a medicine-bonnet, a robe of elk-hide over her shoulders, and elk-teeth on her wrists. The song that she sang when she became a woman was:

"My wristlets are elk-teeth; they are powerful."

Then the woman moved toward a tree, moved her head as if hooking at the tree, and it almost fell. Now when the Elk saw what she was doing, he stopped in great surprise at her power. He did not kill her as he had intended.

This was Elk-Woman. In the sun-dance a tree or post is put up in the centre of the sun-lodge and the woman who wears the bonnet makes hooking motions at the pole, as did the Elk-Woman in the first part of the story.

From Wissler and Duvall (1995), pp. 83–85.

Appendix E: Origin of the Long Time Pipe

I was once camped with my grandfather and father on the Green Banks (St. Mary's River), close to the Rocky Mountains. They were digging out beavers, which were very plentiful. My father went off for a hunt to supply our camp with meat. He followed the trail of some elk up the side of a steep mountain, until he came to timber-line, where he saw a herd of mountain sheep. He followed them towards Nin-ais-tukku (Chief Mountain). When he drew near the summit, he discovered a dense, foul-smelling smoke rising from a deep pit. He pushed a huge boulder into it to hear it fall. There came back no sound, but a cloud of smoke and gas arose so dense and suffocating that he turned to flee, but it was only to meet a black cloud coming up the mountain side. He was frightened and tried to escape, but suddenly there came a terrible crash, and my father fell to the ground. He beheld a woman standing over him. Her face was painted black. Red zig-zag streaks like lightening were below her eyes. Behind the woman stood a man holding a large weapon. My father heard the man exclaim impatiently, "I told you to kill him at once, but you stand there pitying him." He heard the woman chant, "When it rains the noise of the Thunder is my medicine." The man also sang and fired his big weapon. The report was like a deafening crash of thunder, and my father beheld lightning coming from the big hole on the mountain top. He knew nothing more, until he found himself lying inside a great cavern. He had no power to speak, neither could he raise his head, but, when he heard a voice saying, "This is the person who threw the stone down into your fireplace," he realized that he was in the lodge of the Thunder Maker. He heard the beating of a drum, and, after the fourth beating, was able to sit up and look around. He saw the Thunder Chief, in the form of a huge bird, with his wife and many children around him. All of the children had drums, painted with the green talons of the Thunder-bird and with Thunder-bird beaks, from which issued zig-zag streaks of yellow lightning.

We call the thunder Isis-a-kummi (Thunder-bird). We believe that it is a supernatural person. When he leaves his lodge to go through the heavens with the storm-clouds, he takes the form of a great bird with many colours, like the rainbow, and with long green claws. The lightning is the trail of the Thunder-bird.

Whenever the Thunder Maker smoked his pipe, he blew two whiffs upwards towards the sky, and then two whiffs towards the earth. After each whiff, the thunder crashed. Finally the Thunder-bird spoke to my father, saying, "I am the Thunder Maker and my name is Many Drums (expressive of the sound of rolling thunder). You have witnessed my great power and can now go in safety. When you return to your people, make a pipe just like the one you saw me smoking, and add it to your bundle. Whenever you hear the first thunder rolling in the spring-time, you will know that I have come from my cavern, and that it is time to take out my pipe. If you should ever be caught in the midst of a heavy thunder-storm and feel afraid, pray to me, saying, 'Many Drums! Pity me, for the sake of your youngest child,' and no harm will come to you." (This prayer is often used by the Blackfeet during dangerous storms.) As soon as my father returned, he added to his Medicine Bundle a pipe similar to the one shown to him by the Thunder-bird.

From McClintock (1968), pp. 424–26.

Appendix F: Origin of the Medicine Pipe

The Blood Indians have had medicine-pipes for a very long time. There is one pipe among them that is so old that no one has any recollection of having heard of its being made by any one. So this pipe must be the real one handed down by the Thunder, for all medicine-pipes came from the Thunder.

Once there was a girl who never could marry, because her parents could not find any one good enough for her. One day she heard the Thunder roll. "Well," she said, "I will marry him." Not long after this she went out with her mother to gather wood. When they were ready to go home, the girl's packstrap broke. She tied it together and started, but it broke again. Her mother became impatient; and when the strap broke the third time, she said, "I will not wait for you!" The girl started after her mother, but the strap broke again. While she was tying it together, a handsome young man in fine dress stepped out of the brush and said, "I want you to go away with me." The girl said, "Why do you talk to me that way? I never had anything to with you." "You said you would marry me," he answered; "and now I have come for you." The girl began to cry, and said, "Then you must be the Thunder."

Then he told the girl to shut her eyes and not look, and she did so. After a while he told her to look, and she found herself upon a high mountain. There was a lodge there. She went in. There were many seats around the side, but only two people, —an old man and woman. When the girl was seated, the old man said, "That person smells bad." The old woman scolded him, saying that he should not speak thus of his daughter-in-law. Then the old man said, "I will look at her." When he looked up, the lightning flashed about the girl, but did not hurt her. Because of this, the old man knew she belonged to the family. At night all the family came in one by one. The Thunder then made a smudge with sweet-pine needles, one at the door of the lodge, and one just back of the fire. Then he taught his daughter-in-law how to bring in the bundle that hung outside. This was the medicine-pipe. After a time the daughter-in-law gave birth to a boy, later to another boy.

One evening the Thunder asked her if she ever thought of her father and mother. She said that she did. Then he asked would she like to see them. She said, "Yes." So he said, "To-night we will go. You may tell them that I shall send them my pipe, that they may live long." When the time came, he told the woman to close her eyes, and once more she was standing near the lodge of her people. It was dark. She went in and sat down by her mother. After a while she said to her mother, "Do you know me?" "No," was the answer. "I am your daughter. I married the Thunder." The mother at once called in all of their relations. They came and sat around the lodge. The woman told them that she could not stay long as she must go back to her lodge and her children, but that the Thunder would give them his pipe. In four days she would come back with it. Then she went out of the lodge and disappeared.

In four days, the Thunder came with the woman, her two boys, and the pipe. Then the ceremony of transferring the pipe took place. When it was finished, the Thunder said that he was going away, but that he would return in the spring, and that tobacco and berries should be saved for him and prayed over. Then he took the youngest boy and went out. A cloud rolled away, and as it went the people heard one loud thunder and one faint one [the boy]. Now, when the Thunder threatens, the people often say, "For the sake of your youngest child," and he heeds their prayers.

When the Thunder left the woman and elder child behind, he said that if dogs ever attempted to bite them, they would disappear. One day a dog rushed into the lodge and snapped at the boy, after which nothing was seen of him or his mother, and to this day the owner of a medicine-pipe is afraid of dogs.

From Wissler and Duvall (1995), pp. 89–90.

Appendix G: Loss and Capture of the Thunder Pipe

Young Bird Rattle was not his usual, happy self when, late in the afternoon of a day in June, 1879, he came home from hunting with a horseload of buffalo meat. He sat silent, staring at the lodge fire, ate little of the food his mother set before him. She, and the two other wives of his father, Big Bear, kept looking anxiously at him, and at one another, and at last one of them asked if he was sick.

"No, not sick," he shortly answered. And then to me, "Apikuni, go with me to that wise one, Big Elk. It is that I must talk seriously with him."

We found crippled Big Elk sitting upon his couch. His handsome daughter, Ermine Woman, of about 18, upon her couch, sewing a moccasin, shyly looked up at us, bent her head. Bird Rattle had long been one of her unsuccessful suitors. She would not marry because her father needed her constant care, she always said. Big Elk welcomed us, bade us sit, and when he had filled a pipe and passed it to us, Bird Rattle said to him:

Oh, chief, oh, most wise one, while hunting today, I had a strange experience. I saw an eagle standing upon a little hill, pecking, eating something. Seeing me, it flew up, circled above me four times, loudly squawking, then returned to the hill, again pecking, eating what it had there. I neared the hill and the big bird sprang up, winged off southward, again uttering its shrill cries. I found that its food was a raven that it had killed. So, tell me, chief, what was the meaning of it all?

Said Big Elk after long thinking:

Plain enough to me the meaning of that you saw. As you know, returned to us, not long ago, Pine Tree Woman, long a captive of the Crows. She tells me that the one of them, named Raven Calling, whose lodge is painted with a circle of black raven birds, is he who killed my woman, my daughter's loving mother, and got away with my sacred bundle, my sacred Thunder medicine

pipe, and still has it. And now you, named for a bird, a bird's rattle, see an eagle eating a raven; circling above you four times, four the sacred number, and talking to you in its eagle language, and at last flying off southward toward the country of the Crows, and still talking to you. Well, without doubt, my young friend, that was Sun's own way of telling you, and so me, that you are to go after my sacred bundle, and bring it safely back to me.

Said Bird Rattle to that, and at once: "Chief, medicine man of power, that I will try to do, and my friend here, Apikuni, will go with me."

"No, war trail for me. I am a fur trader, nothing else. Come, let us homeward go," I answered.

Bird Rattle was much put out by my refusal to accompany him on his dangerous undertaking. I was in the employ of Joseph Kipp, most successful of the Northwest fur traders, owner of the trading post, Fort Conrad, on the Marias River. I was now on a two-months leave of absence; camping with the Pikuni tribe of the Blackfeet, on the Shonkin Creek; hunting with my close friend, Bird Rattle, and making my home in his father's lodge. That was excitement enough for me.

Early on the following morning, I went up the creek a little way to bathe, and when I returned, Bird Rattle's mother told me that he had been called to Big Elk's lodge. She then gave me a bitter scolding. Her son, she said, was feeling very low because I would not join him in his raid against the Crows. After all he had done for me, twice saved my life, once from being torn apart by a big grizzly that I had wounded, and then from drowning in Big River, how could I refuse to go?

That gave me to think. It was true that, in each instance, he had saved me by his brave and timely help. So, "Oh, cease your fire-talk; do be still," I shortly answered, and when Bird Rattle returned, he was all smiles after I told him that I would go. Saying that we would leave for the Crow country two evenings later, he at once began calling upon some of his friends to join his party.

I had often heard how Big Elk had lost his wife, and his Thunder pipe bundle. Then summers back, when the Pikuni were camping on Sun

River, a number of families of the tribe, wanting some bighorn hides for making thin, soft leather for clothing, set out for the head of Wolf-also-jumped creek (Wolf Creek, between Great Falls and Helena) to kill some of the animals. Well strung out upon the trail, Big Elk and the other men in the lead, their woman following with loaded pack- and travois horses, Big Elk's wife leading a horse carrying his sacred bundle, the party entered the narrow canyon of the creek, and when part way up it, they were suddenly attacked by a war party of Crows that had been following them. Big Elk and all the other men turned back at once, to protect the women as best they could, but the fight was over almost as soon as it began, the Crows making quick retreat after killing five of the party, two men and three women, including Big Elk's wife, and taking the horse that was carrying his sacred bundle. That bundle, it seemed, was the main reason for the Crow's attack, for though they were so many that they could have wiped out the little Pikuni party, they quickly made off with it and were seen no more.

The loss of the Thunder pipe bundle had been a terrible blow, not only to Big Elk, but to the whole Pikuni tribe, for it was believed to have great favour with Sun; to have influenced the great sky god to give good health, good luck to all taking part in its ceremonial rites. Big Elk, soon afterward permanently crippled by a wounded buffalo, had been unable to try to recover the pipe, but a number of war parties of the Pikuni, in that summer and in succeeding summers, had attempted it; but none had done more than kill a few Crows, and make off with a herd of Crow horses. They had, of course, been unable to learn in which one of the more that 300 lodges of the Crow camp the sacred pipe was kept. But now, how different! In a ravens-painted lodge it was, and not much longer to remain there.

Ermine Woman, Big Elk's beautiful daughter, so long his faithful, hard working lodge keeper, was so anxious that the sacred pipe be returned to him that she made a Sun vow that morning. She made the round of the big camp circle, stopping here and there to lift her hands to the sky and chant: "Oh Sun! Oh, powerful traveller of the blue. As you see me, this I vow: Whoever brings my father's sacred Thunder pipe back to him, may have me for his wife.'

Said one of Big Bear's wives to me, after we heard the vow: "See what she is further doing to help her father. She long has loved Bird Rattle. If he be not the one to return the pipe, then must she marry one she does not love, and be ever more unhappy."

During the day, ten of Bird Rattle's friends agreed to join his party, all of them young except Running Wolf, an experienced, successful warrior of about 40 years. He was visiting us, late that evening, planning our route to the Crows, when Big Elk came in, very angry, and said: "Have you heard about Arrow Maker? No? Well, he quietly got together a party to go after my sacred pipe bundle and they have already gone. Yes, gone without having a medicine man give them a going-away sacred sweat, and praying for their success. That means bad luck for them, and possibly for you all, too, as they may get you into serious trouble down in that Crow country."

Said Bird Rattle: "That Arrow Maker. He is doing this because he hates me. Because your daughter is pleasant to me when I visit you, but will not talk with him. He thinks now to get her because of her vow."

"But you can't go before taking the sacred sweat that I am to give you," Big Elk objected.

"You will give it to us early in the morning, and we will then travel fast. So now sleep. To sleep, all of you," said Running Wolf.

On the following morning, we were but five to join Big Elk in the sweat lodge that his daughter and several women helpers had quickly put up for us, the others of our party having backed out because of Arrow Maker's party, already gone. "Well, that need not worry us," Running Wolf said, "for we were going, not to fight the Crows, but to night-seize the sacred bundle and make off with it, and for that, the fewer we were, the better." So, wrapped only in our blankets, we entered the little enclosure, thrust the blankets out under the lodgeskin, and naked sat. The women passed in some redhot rocks; we rolled them into a pit in the centre of the lodge; Big Elk, singing a song to Sun, dipped a buffalo tail in a dish of water, sprinkled them, and at once dense steam enveloped us and we began to sweat. It fairly dripped from us as he prayed for our safety and success. Ermine Woman passed in a lighted pipe, and in turn we smoked it as we prayed the Above Ones to keep us safe in all that we were to do, the ceremony ending by Big Elk saying that he would daily pray for us. We reached out for our blankets, and, wrapped in them, ran to the creek and bathed in the cool water. We hurried to our lodges to dress and prepare to leave.

All that day, we travelled as fast as we could walk, southeastward across the plain. At dusk, after a short rest, hurried on again until, at midnight, and worn out, we struck Arrow Creek and slept. Came morning, and we killed a deer, broiled and ate some of it, and were off again. Herds of buffalo and bands of antelope were everywhere in sight; grazing, resting, in long files going to water, and from it. We could not avoid frightening a herd now and then, and that made us nervous; their flight was a plain call to any enemy war party that might be thereabouts, to come and fall upon us. With all the power of the Blackfeet language, we denounced Arrow Maker for obliging us to run such risk. But for him we would be travelling only at night, leisurely and unafraid.

Pine Tree Woman had said that we would find the Crows camped somewhere up Bighorn River, so we were heading to cross the Yellowstone at the mouth of that river, and follow it up. Therefore, on direct route to it, we had our next short rest and sleep on Judith River, and near sunset of our third day out, nearing Armell's Creek, decided to rest in its well-timbered valley until midnight. As we were entering the timber, we were startled by hearing, close on our left, someone cry out: "Ha! More Pikuni men arrive!" And out from a clump of willows came Fox Eyes, a member of Arrow Maker's party. He said that the others were in by the creek, preparing to eat, and led us to them. They had just started a fire and were sitting around it, nine of them, and all got up with pleasant words of greeting, all save Arrow Maker. He only glanced at us, then began putting more sticks upon the fire. That made his men uneasy;

they stopped talking; looked at one another, and down at him. Then said Running Wolf: "Arrow Maker, it is no wonder that you keep your head down; well you know that you have no right to go after Big Elk's Thunder pipe."

"Why haven't I that right?" he asked.

"Because he appointed Bird Rattle to attempt to get it."

"That matters not to me," bold-faced and hard-eyed Arrow Maker growled. "The sacred bundle is for anyone who can take it from the Crows. I shall do my utmost to be that one."

Said Running Wolf:

"Arrow Maker, I advise you not to attempt it; for Sun, in his own, sacred way, made it known to Big Elk that Bird Rattle should go for it." And with that, went on to tell of the latter's experience with the raven. He finished, and said one of the other part, Little Otter: "Ha, we did not know that. Surely Bird Rattle is the one for this sacred undertaking. It is not for us to interfere."

"Matters not to me, all this about the raven. I have set out to get that sacred bundle. Get it I shall, and for it, get the woman that I want," said Arrow Maker, and angrily.

At that, Bird Rattle, shouting, "Oh, you dog-face!" made to step forward, but Running Wolf and I seized and held him, as several of Arrow Maker's men laid hold of him, prevented him reaching for his gun.

Said Bird Rattle: "I was wrong. Sun is against us Pikuni fighting one another. Let us move on."

While taking off our moccasins to wade the creek, we heard loud talk of those we had left around their fire. We crossed the stream, had not gone far when Little Otter overtook us, asked if he could join our party? Bird Rattle answered that we would be glad to have him with us. Then asked why the loud talk that we had heard. Well, it was that two of the party had urged Arrow Maker to turn back home, as they believed that Sun was not in favour of their undertaking. Arrow Maker had replied that his medicine was much more powerful than that of Bird Rattle; he was going on, and would, himself, take the sacred bundle from the Crows. Then, without another word, the two had taken up their belongings and turned back for home.

No more was said until, well out from Armell's Creek, we stopped for a short rest, and to eat some broiled meat that we had carried from our previous stop. We had done well to overtake the party in so short a time, but still had a hard task before us; it was to travel all the night; and with short rests, keep on going in order to be first to strike the Crow camp. From this point, there were two ways, of about equal length, to strike the mouth of the Bighorn; by crossing the gap in the mountains at the head of Armell's Creek; by rounding the north end of Snowy Mountains. Little Otter said that Arrow Maker was going through the gap, so we took to the other course.

Near sunset, three days later, we struck the Yellowstone, about a mile above the mouth of the Bighorn. Though so tired that we fairly ached, still we must keep going. We killed a buffalo, ate, and broiled enough more of its meat to last several days. By this time, night was come, but we managed to find a big pile of driftwood on a sandbar, and made a raft of light, dry logs that we pulled from it, lashing them together with rawhide ropes that we carried. Then piling our clothing, weapons, various belongings upon the raft, we put out into the stream, hanging to its sides and rear end, and paddling and kicking, did our best to force it toward the other shore.

But the current was swift and contrary. Twice it forced us into the side from which we had started, and when at last we did make the other shore, we were all of a mile below the mouth of the Bighorn, and so chilled, exhausted, that we trembled as we got out clothes, and lay down to rest, in Crow country at last.

Bird Rattle had us all up before dawn, and when day came we were heading up the valley of the Bighorn, keeping well within the timber bordering its shore. As there were no buffalo nor antelope in sight, we thought that the Crow camp might be near, and were made certain of it when, after an hour or so of travel, we saw herds of horses upon the east slope of the valley. As we stood staring at them, a sudden outburst of angry, fighting dogs warned us that we were almost upon the camp, much too near it, and we ran through the grove, and into a thick growth of willows a few yards from the river. Soon after we had dropped down in them, a number of women came chattering along from camp and began gathering wood for their lodges. We all lay flat upon the ground, not daring to lift our heads to look at them. For a time, two worked quite near us, talking as they chopped dry branches and made bundles of them. Great was our relief when they all turned back campward with their loads.

That was a long and trying day, for we were in constant risk of discovery by wood gatherers, and children playing along the shore of the river. Came night.

We went out to the shore, drank, ate some of our broiled meat. Worried about Arrow Maker; feared that he and his men could not be far off. Then Bird Rattle gave us his plan for taking the sacred bundle. First, we would look for the ravens-painted lodge. Having found it, we would catch horses for our getaway, and while our companions held them all in readiness, he and I could slip into the lodge, seize the bundle and run. He, himself, would cut the bundle from the lodgepole to which it was undoubtedly tied, and it was for me to prevent the lodge man interfering with him. That didn't please me at all. I was about to object, say that I did not want to fight a Crow, even if he had killed one or two Pikuni when taking the bundle. But to my relief, up spoke Running Wolf, claiming that privilege. Said he: "Bird Rattle, I, not Apikuni, am the one to go into that lodge with you and kill the Crow therein, for as you know, he, or one of his party, killed my mother's sister when they seized the sacred bundle."

"As you say. You, then," Bird Rattle answered shortly, and led off up the grove. We soon threaded our way to its end, and there before us, in a wide, long grassy reach of the valley, and plain in the moonlight, was the big Crow camp, a circle ten or fifteen lodges in width, and a quarter of a mile in diameter. The lodges were dimly glowing with the fires within them. Men and women were going from lodge to lodge; visiting; feasting; drumming; singing; talking and laughing. It would be long until they would tire, and sleep. So we sat on and on, watching the camp, watching our rear, fearing to see Arrow Maker and his party appear.

The freed-from-the-Crows Pikuni woman had said that the ravens-painted lodge always stood in the north side of the camp circle, but when, near midnight, we made sure that it was not there, we thought that she had been mistaken in its location, so made the whole round of the camp and found that there was no such lodge in it. So, what to do? "Naught to do but to round up a big band of Crow horses and make off with them," said Little Otter. "But," said Bird Rattle: "You see that many of the lodgeskins are of new, white leather, as though but yesterday sewn together and put up. It may be that the lodge we seek is such a one, and has not yet been raven-painted. We must wait a night or two, on the chance that it may be done."

Said Running Wolf: "Ha! I noticed on this north side of the camp a sweat lodge covered with pieces of old lodge skins. Wait you here, I will see if any of them are raven-painted."

We had not long to wait. He returned, stepping high and smiling. Said that, sure enough, the coverings were parts of the old raven-painted lodge skin. Without doubt, one of the new white lodges near it would soon be raven-painted, and it was for us to be patient and wait for it.

"Ha! Wait and starve. Not good," one growled.

"Wait for that Arrow Maker party to arrive and get us into trouble," said another.

Said Bird Rattle: "Go any of you, all of you, if you so feel about it. Myself, I came here for that sacred bundle, and shall do my best to get it."

"Nor shall we starve, though we dare not hunt. Plenty of drying meat in that camp for our taking of it," said Running Wolf.

That was so. Here and there between the lodges were high-strung lines of buffalo meat, cut into thin sheets to dry for future use, or for making pemmican. Our two dissatisfied companions having ceased to growl, we all stole in to take some of it, so I, for the first time, entered an enemy camp. We moved slowly, noiselessly, often pausing to look and listen. Standing so close to a lodge that we could hear the breathing of some heavy sleeper in it. I, anyhow, fearful that at any

moment, someone would come from a lodge and see us, set the whole camp upon us. We came to a tightly-strung rawhide rope upon which many sheets of meat were drying, well above the reach of the camp dogs, and when we had taken all that we could handily carry of it, Bird Rattle cut the rope, then frayed the ends against a stone, so rubbing out the neat, smooth knife cut; making it appear that the rope had broken of itself, and that the dogs had devoured the meat. We then stole out of the camp, and hurrying down the valley for a mile or more, turned into the timber, built a fire, roasted and ate a lot of the meat, and slept.

Up at dawn, we moved deep into the willows close to the river, to pass the day, a day of restless worrying for us all. Mainly about the Arrow Maker party. As we had seen nothing of them, believed that, in crossing the Yellowstone, they had managed to land above the mouth of the Bighorn, and coming up the opposite side of it, and discovering the Crow camp, they were like us, in hiding somewhere near it, intent on finding the ravens-painted lodge. Well, there was but one thing to do. Keep on with our plan to get the sacred bundle just as though they were not also after it. Like the Pikuni, and all plains tribes, the Crows brought in their fast buffalo horses every evening and picketed them closely before the lodges. Come night, and we should find the lodge we sought, they were the horses that we would take for our get-away.

No Crows came near us that day. Nor did we hear any of them moving about. We had fine weather, clear sunny days so far, but now, as evening came on, a cool north wind set in, and the sky clouded over, threatening rain. That pleased our leaders. Sun was with us, helping us, they said. Far better darkness than moonlight for what we were to do.

Came time for us to go, and as we were taking up our belongings, Bird Rattle said to us: "Now, my friends, one last thing. There is no knowing what may happen to us up there. Should we become separated, get into trouble, let it be understood that here, right here, will be our meeting place."

So again we approached the Crow camp, its many lodges glowing redly with the fires within them. We had come too early, but Bird Rattle had insisted on it, saying that he could not wait to learn if one of the new lodges had been ravens-painted. Halting us at a safe distance from the camp, he went on alone. After a time, he came hurrying back, exclaiming: "It is there, my friends, it is there, the lodge we seek. It stands at the outer edge of this north part of the circle."

"Good! Good! Soon, with Sun's help, shall I be killing my mother's sister's killer," said Running Wolf.

We had to wait long for the camp to quiet down, the lodge fires die out, the people sleep. The clouds were thinning, the darkness lightening when Bird Rattle said

Let us begin. Best that we do not go together. Little Otter, New Robe, Young Bull, you three turn into the camp farther up. Apikuni, you come with Running Wolf and me. If all goes well, we will meet right here with our takings of horses, and then try to get the sacred bundle. But if trouble comes and we are scattered, remember that we meet where we stopped below.

Said Running Wolf:

Mind this, you youngsters: Do not attempt to take a horse whose rope goes into a lodge. That is a well-known trick of a Crow—fastening the end of the rope to his ankle or wrist and now and then pulling on it to learn if his horse is still there.

Bird Rattle leading, I close following Running Wolf, we slowly, noiselessly neared the ravens-painted lodge. I could see four of the big, black bird paintings upon its new, white leather skin. The sky had now cleared, the moon was brightly shining. That was bad. I had looked for the darkness to protect us in all that we were to do. I had a strange, stifling feeling of coming trouble as we stepped nearer to the side of the lodge. How crazy I had been to come upon this sacred bundle quest. Oh, never again. Never again. Running Wolf nudged me, and turned my attention to Bird Rattle, and he pointed to some horses standing

before lodges to our left, signed that we would go to them. But just as we were starting, a gun boomed in the river side of the camp circle, then another one, and as men began yelling and running that way from their lodges, Bird Rattle said to Running Wolf: "Come quick. Our only chance to get it!"

Well, I was not going to be left alone out there. As we ran to the doorway of that ravens-painted lodge, so did Arrow Maker, coming from we knew not where, and thrusting Bird Rattle back to be first in. Bird Rattle seized him, said to him: "Go back! Not for you, the sacred bundle." But Arrow Maker broke loose, dived in through the doorway, and we close followed. In there, as in all the other lodges, women and children were chattering and shrieking with fear, for over in the other side of the camp, men were still yelling and shooting. But the man of this lodge had not gone and, angrily roaring, he crushed Arrow Maker's skull with a blow of his war club, and would have killed Bird Rattle, coming next had he not parried the blow with the barrel of his gun. Then, before he could again raise the war club, Running Wolf stabbed him deep in the breast, and even as he fell, Bird Rattle was cutting the sacred bundle loose from a lodgepole at the head of the man's couch, and saying to us: "I have it. We go."

"Not until I get this," answered Running Wolf, bending over the lodge man and taking his scalp, there before his women and children, now silent, paralyzed with fear.

As we ran out into the bright moonlight, a nearby woman saw us and ran shouting for help. It was us for the timber as fast as we could go, and the shouts of men taking after us was loud in our ears. But as they had gathered at the far side of camp, we had a long start of them, and gaining the timber, we sped down in it to our meeting place, where our companions anxiously awaited our coming. They had not even entered the camp when the firing began. Stopping only to regain our breath, we hurried on down the valley to the Yellowstone and hearing nothing of our enemies, built another raft and recrossed it. Day was just breaking when we landed, and taking out rope lashings, let the raft logs drift away.

There was mourning in camp when, ten days later, we came to it on the Shonkin, for only three of Arrow Maker's party had returned. Like us, he had discovered the ravens-painted lodge and had made his men to pretend to attack the river side of the camp, so to give him the chance to slip into the lodge and take the sacred bundle, with the result that the Crows had responded to the attack so quickly, and in such numbers, that in the retreat, three of Arrow Maker's party had been killed, the others escaping only by swimming the Bighorn.

But Big Elk was happy in having gotten back his sacred Thunder pipe; Ermine Woman in having at last the one man whom she wanted, and Bird Rattle in having her. On an evening when I was visiting them, he said to me: "Apikuni, what happiness, what excitement that was, our taking of the sacred bundle. We must go to war; have more of it."

"Never again. Never again. From now on, I shall be a trader, nothing more," I answered.

From Schultz, 1936.

Appendix H:
Transfer History of the Small Medicine Thunder Pipe

My Pipe came from Browning. Someone named Sooiee made it. He transferred the Pipe to Fish Wolf Robe (Mamii'owa), both were living in Browning. My parents, Willy Crowshoe and his wife All-Listen-To (Ikisanopa), the later Mrs. Buffalo (in second marriage), went to Browning to ask for the pipe, the Small Pipe, from Fish Wolf Robe. But Mamii'owa had just given the pipe to a man from Siksika. He had promised the pipe already to Good Chaser. Fish Wolf Robe gave the pipe as a gift to Good Chaser from Gleichen. Good Chaser didn't pay for it; it was given. Good Chaser transferred it to Hind Bull from the Bloods. He transferred it to Many Chiefs from Brocket, and then it went in transfer to Many Feathers, Nathan Many Feathers, also from Brocket. The Old Man Awakasina and the Old Lady then got it transferred from the Old Man Many Feathers. When my dad Willy Crowshoe, Deer Chief (Awakasina), was gone the Old Lady kept the Pipe and my dad's brother came and said "I want to take my brother's pipe." But the Old Lady said, "No, I still use it; the pipe has his home here. I will keep it."

I was still young then but the Old Lady told me to take the pipe because her husband (Joe Buffalo) did not care about it. I was staying somewhere else because I was not comfortable there.

Where I slept I had a dream of a person who came and said, "Come and get me." I dreamed the same dream the next night. That morning I saddled up my horse and told my mom. She said it was the Pipe talking and I should come and get it. The next morning I put up my horses and the buggy and drove up to mother's house. She smudged and prayed with me and then we brought the Pipe home.

I have had the pipe since then and take care of it. Every spring I spend all the money on my Pipe. Today, I am still having a Pipe dance. Look here, I didn't get it for nothing; it was hard to get it; the same with the other things that were given to me. We should tell the whole story. The same with my Buffalo Hoof Tipi when it was given to me in Gleichen at the Sundance.

Joe Crowshoe (1997)

Appendix I:
Interview: Bull Horn Doctor

Now these are the story I have being telling you about. The one I told about healed me, I seen him and this one I am going to tell about, I seen him too, he is my grandfather. His name is Holy Come Down. That was his name. He was really old. I think it might have been sixty years since he died. He was still a very young boy then. I think it was seventy years, nearly seventy years since he died. He was 97 when he died, just three more years to make a 100.

He was alone when they went to war. They fled; he had a horse which he got from the enemy. He went off by himself up a mountain. He went along the edge leading this horse he got when it slipped and fell into the gully. Its feet were up. He was flat on his back. He couldn't get him on his feet so he left him and fled. He didn't know where his comrades went. He didn't bother going any place. He just stayed up on that mountain. Where he was to flee there was no shelter, like trees, so he stayed up on that mountain. He stayed up there all day. That night he went back to the enemy camp. A horse was tied in front; he jump on it and ran off, not knowing it was a real fast horse. He was chased but couldn't catch him. So there he was walking. At daylight he came to this gully. There he tied this horse, pulling grass and put it by him. He got a lot for him, then he went off to hide elsewhere. If the horse was found he will not be found by him. Where he hide he cried and prayed not to be found. Finally he fell asleep because he had been running all night. He fell asleep with the heat of the day. In his sleep he seen this man. It told him "Son come." Then he seen this lone buffalo sitting there. These lone buffalo are old bulls. It was going to heal himself. Then he seen it become a man and this man that came to him told him, "I am going to heal him." That's why I went to get you to look. He seen this buffalo man sitting there with his leg broken in four places. The man sang for himself. He said, "If tomorrow comes; if I make it to the next day nothing will happen to me." The buffalo said to this man, "If we are real hungry and make it to the next day nothing happens to us." This was in the man's dream. Then this man told him, "I am going to heal him, the buffalo with the broken leg." He took a bag with a weasel in it. This man seen all this in his dream and the buffalo had seen this thing about the weasel in his dream too.

The weasel was held on the broken part and was blown on. When blown on it stood up. Four times it was blown on and four times it stood up. Then this man told the buffalo, "I am powerful. In four days you will walk on this leg." The grass is sweet grass. That was what he used. The weasel, that day, had the head pointing down when tied onto the leg. The next day as he was going to change the dressing, the weasel's head was pointing up. It had turned. So yellow paint was used on it again the weasel. Again the head was put pointing down. The next day when it was unwrapped, it had turn again, head pointing upward. The dressing used was sweet grass. This time, the head of the weasel was put upward, and the next day when unwrapped it had turned, head pointing downward. The leg had not swelled anymore. The weasel was tied tight when put on. How did it manage to turn downward or upward every time?

It told him, "My son, this I give you." Then he woke up, it was getting dark. Where he had walked there was some sweet grass. He took some and chewed on it. That was his meal and he got home safely. That's when he got himself a weasel skin. That was the weasel he seen.

There is this man that just died. His name was Big Sorrel Horse. He had a slight limp. His leg was broken below the knees. It had turned bad, it was full of pus and smelled. They came for my grandfather to heal him. He went. The fourth day, he was able to walk. I didn't see how he did it. But it was later when Big Sorrel Horse told me about it, the way my grandfather healed him. It was said, these old people telling the story said, that man's leg was poisoned and how powerful was he that healed him. A weasel he used and every time unwrapped it had turned.

"My father Little White Calf was drunk. From the wagon buckboard he jumped off it. His leg got into the wheel and broke just below the knee. They went for his father to heal him. When he looked at it, his father said your leg had been touched, if it was not touched, it will not be more than four days you will walk again. He took some sweet grass, first chewed it, then sprayed the leg with it. In his dream, he had put the bone in place. He had the weasel skin facing up and then it was tied. There was not sticks to tie it with; it was just tied like that. The next day, the nights are counted. The next day when unwrapped the weasel was facing downward. The dressing was put on with the weasel facing upward. The next day, it was facing down. Then it was put facing down, the next day when unwrapped it was facing up. So it was put down again, and the next day it was facing upward again. Then it was taken away. My father walked in twenty-seven days. He didn't have a limp. It was my father's father. When he was dying, Holy Come Down, he told my father I will paint you on it. Take the weasel, with yellow paint he used on his forehead slanting it to the right. And his hands, yellow was painted on the back of the hand and that was the weasel given to my father.

He had the weasel. This man called George Big Wolf had a broken leg. My father healed him. He used dry skin to wrap the leg and tied it, having the weasel facing upward. The next day, when he unwrapped it, it was facing downward. My father was glad. He put it on again. It was not his dream, it was given to him in ceremony. When he put it on again, he had it facing upward, and when unwrapped the next day, it was facing downward again. The next day, he changed it around the other way, facing down. These four days, two days he had it facing upwards and two days he had it facing downward. His name was Bonnie and he walked. He just died not too long ago.

This one had a broken arm; his name was Three Persons, Good Offering. Just above the elbow was where the arm broke and my father healed him. It is very hard because it is not his dream. It was his father's dream, and he was the one that gave him the healing powers. He had the weasel facing upward. He didn't change the dressing often, just once a day. The next day, when he unwrapped it, the weasel was facing downward. He was just glad because the weasel had moved.

The next day, when he looked at it, it had changed position. He was really glad the next day; when he looked at it again, it was facing down. The next day, it was facing up. So he was just being glad. He put it facing down again. The next day when he checked it, it was facing upward, and that was the last day. It took him twenty-seven days to be back on his feet again; he was alright then.

My father knew then that his healing was real good. He had others, his own dreams. It was said he was very powerful with his healing. What was given to him in ceremony he was using to save people.

Myself, I went to get the horses, these rain shoes I had on, was getting summer. It was in the Spring, the horse I rode stepped in a hole and fell and I felled too, breaking my leg just below the knee. It broke in three. I didn't lay out there long, maybe an hour, before someone found me. They brought a sleigh which they put me on to carry me home. My father told me "to try hard, that it was easy to set the bone right." I took a towel, rolled it and bit it. There is Good Do, Good Doo his name is many-plaited hair. He held me down at the midsection and my mother held the other leg. I seen my father use sage on his hands then seen him lean down. I couldn't see because this man was laying in front. I just felt hold my leg and he straightened it. I blacked out when he did this. The towel I had in my mouth, I bit on it hard; I didn't know. When I came back to, cold water was being used on my face and head. My leg was straightened by then, and the weasel was wrapped with the leg. Those cardboard boxes, that was the kind of paper used to wrap my leg. They just put some padding around the leg. I had it up and my father was doctoring me himself. When he had finished doing this, I felt good and slept. When I woke up, it was getting dark. The next day, my father unwrapped it. This was the second time he fixed it. My father he had a dog tail. He healed me with the dogs. He just licked my leg. When he did this, my leg felt good. It didn't hurt. He used sweet grass on it. It was broken in three places. When he finished, he wrapped it again with the weasel.

The next day was when he was going to change it. I never felt anything that night, but the next day when he checked it, it had turned facing down. My father was glad. He fixed it again, and I went back to sleep. When I am falling asleep, I happen to move somehow. I just cry because my leg hurted. The next day when my leg was checked, it had faced down. The next day, it face down. The next day, it faced up. Twice it faced down, twice it face up.

Then my father said I am not powerful if over thirty days with the broken leg. Then he sang a word song. That song they heard. If I make it to the next day, nothing happens. That was the song he sang. That's where he finished looking after me. Twenty days after, I got up using crutches. Twenty-seven days after, my leg broke again, the same leg and from a horse, too. It was the same dog that he healed me with. Today when my leg healed, there are no scars on it.

Just lately, it was the same leg just at the ankle it broke again. There is this son of mine called Clive; he had a broken leg too. My father healed Clive. In four days, he walked. That was the weasel. When he did, I took the weasel. There was no holy things given to me. That son of mine, that fighter Edward, he broke his arm. I just tied the weasel with his arm. Just at the muscle; that's

where it broke, so I tied it with the weasel facing up. The next day, when I untied it, it had turned. The next day, it faced down. So I put it facing down. It was up the next day. I put it facing down again, and the next day was the final day when I checked it, it was facing up. My son's broken arm—right now he is over there—it had no scar. It was not given to me, but I saved it.

I left these things of mine with Brown just for a while. I didn't know he would do this. All of these things of mine he took and sold them all. He sold with the weasel and that bear claw. If he hadn't sold it, I would still have it. These are the things I saw. Like myself with my broken leg, there was no scar. That's how amazing Indian way of life is. If we can just believe in it, we can use it. That's what these are that I am telling about. There are many that I will tell about. I will tell them as far as I know them. These are what I seen a broken leg that's why I showed them. They were not given to me in the holy way. It is just with my good thinking that I gave the person what he got better with.

This is where I finish telling of the broken legs and arms.

That's all.

Interviewed by Marie Waterchief (no date)

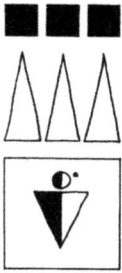

Notes

Chapter 1

1 Chapter 5 on Transfer Rites will describe how "authorization" is understood and can be achieved in traditional Blackfoot culture.

2 The term "medicine" is often used to describe the healing or curing applications of these powers.

3 This model can be regarded as a management tool in areas other than health and can be applied by groups other than Peigan, even non-Native communities. It is an option for management structures on the same level as other formats.

4 Not only does this process of selection happen when "original" information is collected, but additional selections take place when these data are recorded, published, and presented orally (Berreman 1968, p. 339).

5 Although anyone's observations are biased by social role, upbringing, particular professional endeavours, and one's understanding of oneself in relation to another culture, the researchers want to emphasize that because these first white men came from a specific stratum in Victorian society with very specific intentions, their background coloured the way they talked about the Blackfoot people.

6 For example, Palliser (Spry 1963) usually mentions the Kootenays and Stoneys in a better light than the Blackfoot he encounters. He mentions their cleanliness, their willingness to help the expedition, and their conversion to Christianity: "On now taking leave of the Kootanies, with whom I have been camped for nearly a week, it is but justice to say, that they behaved in a very civil and hospitable manner; and although our clothes and other articles have been lying about in all directions, we have (with the exception of some hide lines, moccasins, and other articles of leather, which the half-starved dogs have eaten) not lost a single article.... Whether this honesty is attributed of the knowledge of Christianity spread among them by the ministers of the Roman Catholic church, or whether it is innate in them, I can only say that it is a great contrast to the effect produced by the missions in the Indian territory on the east side," p. 173).

7 This has recently been argued by several authors in relation to the signing of the treaties (Ray 1996, Taylor 1987). (See also Chapter 2.)

8 "We know now that individuals use memory the way scientists use data, which is to say that people scan their past, as well as their present, for information that will confirm what they already know or strongly suspect. At the same time, what they already know and expect significantly influences what they will see and remember. In oversimplified terms, what we remember of the past molds the present, while what we are concerned with in the present shapes our memory of the past" (Baur 1991, p. 190).

Chapter 2

1 The North West Mounted Police, who later became the Royal Canadian Mounted Police, met the first Blackfoot Nation members in August, 1874, at present-day Fort Walsh (Denny 1972, Dunn 1994, Steele 1915). Since the NWMP's settlement in Fort Macleod in October 1874, there were ongoing and regular meetings with the North Peigan, Blood, and Blackfoot (Macleod 1931, Nevitt 1974).

2 These are usually published manuscripts or unpublished field notes that date from the reservation period and include Blackfoot people's memories of pre-reservation years. Foremost ethnographers on the South and North Peigan are Duvall/Wissler, McClintock, Schultz, and Ewers.

3 Interviews accessed for this research exist in transcribed form and are located in the Old Man River Cultural Centre in Brocket on the Peigan Reserve, the Glenbow Museum Archives in Calgary, and the Provincial Museum Archives in Edmonton.

4 Primarily David Charles Duvall (1910, 1911), Percy Bullchild (1985), and Mike Mountain Horse (1979).

5 The dog and horse days are also often termed as the buffalo days and are characterized by dependency on hunting the buffalo, either by buffalo jumps or pounds and, in later times, with the use of the horse.

6 See Appendix A, "Creation Story."

7 Kelsey (1929) might have been the first white man who met Blackfoot between 1691 and 1692 on the southern Saskatchewan prairies. However, this meeting is questioned by some historians.

8 Archaeologists have explored various bison kill sites that are scattered over the prairies and can be dated back 11,000 years. They describe the elaborate systems developed by the people and the effectiveness of these techniques (Brink 1992, Ewers 1949,).

9 "The people have no other medicine to lead buffalo over the drive or make them come, outside of the story of the woman who first found the Buffalo rock. When buffalo are far away the Buffalo rocks and songs are used to bring them near. The Black Buffalo painted lodge is used to bring the buffalo near as they have the Buffalo rocks, the Beaver men get the buffalo hoofs from the Buffalo lodge owners ... the woman who found the buffalo rock was married to a man who owned a beaver bundle. This woman gave her rocks to the Buffalo lodge owners" (Red Plume, in Duvall 1911).
See also Wissler and Duvall (1995, pp. 85-89) on three different versions of the Buffalo Rock.

10 See Chapter 4 on the meaning of bundles.

11 By 1754, Anthony Henday (1907) possibly met Blackfoot, who had guns and horses and regarded them as "good horsemen." In 1772, Matthew Cocking (1908) already reported on the three different divisions of the Blackfoot. However, all three Blackfoot tribes shared the same language and customs. They were politically independent divisions, with the primary social organization in bands and occasional seasonal tribal gatherings.

12 Alexander Culbertson and David Mitchell were the first American Fur Company employees who started trade with the Blackfoot people at Fort McKenzie. James Kipp came to Fort Union in 1831 after a peace treaty was signed with Blackfoot and Assiniboine. Culbertson later married Medicine Snake, a Blood woman who was a sister of Seen from Afar (Ewers 1962).

13 For example, Blackfoot traditional values really changed because of the introduction of liquor. The appearance of whisky and trading posts (Fort Whoop-Up, Fort Kipp, Fort Slide Out) prompted some Blackfoot men to force their women to work as prostitutes for fort employees in Fort Macleod and Lethbridge. (Gray 1971).

14 In 1879, the count of North Peigan people who had settled on the Peigan reserve was about 900 (Department of Indian Affairs 1880).

15 There is clear evidence that North Peigan chiefs did not understand the terms and consequences of their signing the treaty. Some authors (Ray 1996, Taylor 1987) have argued that this was based on a lack of proper translation, but also that the Native leaders were misled into believing that they were signing a peace treaty rather than surrendering their traditional lands and restricting their movements. (In exchange for "making

peace," they would receive monies and provisions, education for their children, and health care). Aside from these central misconceptions, the way the Canadian government (primarily the Department of Indian Affairs) chose to interpret the general tone of the treaty was based on Western thinking and was totally different from what the Peigan understood they had agreed to. For example, the two understand the concepts of land use and land occupation entirely differently. Some Peigan elders said they were told "that they were going to have a better life, if they made the treaty ... and that they were promised education, medical assistance, money and to be rid of whiskey traders" (Hildebrandt 1996).

16 Although there might have been some agents who had the interest of the Native population at heart (see Wilson's 1921 letter of protest regarding the treatment of Blood tribe members: "Our Betrayed Wards"), other agents were abusive and fraudulent, using their power to enrich themselves by selling or leasing land illegally to settlers and pocketing the money personally. The same can be said for the sale of cows, farming equipment, and agricultural products, where the agent either took a cut or kept all the money. Agents gave preferential allotment of jobs and medical care to "favourites" and controlled the movements of residents through a "pass system." They had total control over their "fiefdom" and decision-making power over nearly all aspects of reserve life.
Raczka (1979) gives the following chronological list of Indian agents for the North Peigan: C. Kettles, White Beard, C. Kettles, Sorrel Whiskers, Irving, Springet, Pocklington, Mr. Naste (?), R.N. Wilson (left 1907), G.H. Gooderham, E.H. Yeomans, H.A. Guin (1913), I.H. Graham (1918), and A.O. Arthur (p. 91). North Peigan elders remember different names and time frames: Pocklington (1882), Wilson (1898 to 1911), Graham (1921), and Nash; and, from 1938 on, Lancaster, Faunt, Hunter, Woodsworth, and Cousneau (interviews with Peigan elders, Oldman River Cultural Centre, Brocket).

17 As the government was scared of a potential new Riel Rebellion, a pass system was introduced to control movement: "In 1886 the government introduced this shameful scheme, which required Plains Indians to carry passes for all off-reservation activities. To obtain a pass, a person had to get the approval of the local farming instructor and the Indian agent who issued the passes, which gave these officials dictatorial control over the lives of Indians. Agents denied passes to anyone they thought was troublesome, and the police backed them up by patrolling the borders of the reserves day and night looking for absentees. In this way, Indian Affairs essentially imprisoned Native people in reserves" (Ray 1996, p. 233). Even to be able to dance in their authentic costumes off the reserve in any public affair, Indians needed permission from the Indian agent (Doucet, no date Ray 1996).

18 With the signing of Treaty 7, North Peigan/ Blackfoot people gained the right to "white man's" education for their children. This led to the establishment of Roman Catholic (Father Scollen) and Anglican (Reverend Haynes) missions on the Peigan reserve, and Methodist and Presbyterian churches on other Blackfoot reserves. Haynes arrived in 1879, but the Catholic missionaries seemed to have settled earlier on the north side of the Old Man River. In 1887, a Roman Catholic church (Sacred Heart) and school were started at the Old Agency, and, in 1888, an Anglican school (St. Cyprian's) was founded on the south side of the river.

19 For example, the important time in the summer to celebrate the Sun Dance as a religious as well as a central social activity was the time when farming activities were supposed to happen. Indian agents and farm instructors who wanted their "charges" to hay rather than spend weeks in the Sun Dance camp forbade the Sun Dance. In an 1895 amendment to the Indian Act, the Sun Dance was forbidden, based on elements that involved self-torture. The agents, with the help of the NWMP, tried to stop the ritual. In the face of these threats, some tribes changed their ritual and left their children in the residential missionary schools.

20 The Anglicans started a boarding school in 1890, called Victoria Home, and the Catholics followed in 1896. Some elders remember different dates for the beginning of the boarding school era on Peigan land. Other dates given are 1909 and 1904 for the Anglican school. Federal subsidies by the Department of Indian Affairs were paid per student to the schools, but they did not cover all costs, and often other congregations made contributions. Also, students often spent more than half of their school hours doing manual labour to provide food for themselves and their teachers.

21 In 1920, Indian Affairs decided to force parents to send their children to school, which meant that all aboriginal children between seven and fifteen years of age attended Indian schools. Most children who went to the local residential schools entered at a very early age (between four and six years of age) and experienced culture shock, punishment, and abuse, were made ashamed of their heritage, and received a mostly substandard level of education (North Peigan elders interviews). Additionally, we know of health problems in these schools; they were a breeding ground for tuberculosis and other diseases. The last of these Indian residential schools in Canada was closed in 1988.

22 Figures were often calculated on the basis of number of tipis and these were multiplied by estimated number of inhabitants. For example, Dempsey (1988) gives these population estimates:

23 For example, Manneschmidt (1994), in her research with the Kham Magar, a tribal group of people in the Himalayas, describes how malnutrition and extreme physical strain had a strong effect on women's fertility. Other research (Frisch 1974, Frisch et al. 1975) shows how a certain amount of body fat in women is a prerequisite for ovulation. One can assume that consecutive years of starvation had a strong impact on Blackfoot women's fertility.

24 But 1842, 1876, and 1904 were years when horses died, and 1886, 1891, and 1909 when cattle died, a situation which must have affected the North Peigan's food supplies.

25 Jenness (1955) mentions that 600 Blackfoot died of starvation just after the disappearance of the buffalo.

26 The Government of Canada knew in 1879 about the severity of the situation, but lack of logistics and money led to little action by federal politicians.

Chapter 3

1 A Mrs. Wadsworth (1968) from the Blood Reserve was married when she was seven years old and her husband was eleven years older. Sixty-five years later, she related how her parents would rig up a travois, pack bedding, food, clothing, and blankets, and load a horse with extra gifts to take to her future in-laws.

2 The first wife usually stayed in the most central position in the tipi on the eastern side. She was called the "Sits Beside Wife," thus ensuring her dominant position in the household.

3 In many other Native groups, the term "clan" is used to describe the same kind and size of social unit. However, most of these groups use totemic names to describe their affiliations – a method not used in Blackfoot culture.

4 De Josselin de Jong (1912) argues, based on his field work and linguistic research, that marriages were exogamous in relation to band membership.

5 Dempsey describes how "a band of the Bloods called Followers of the Buffalo kept growing in size because of its wise leadership, and every few years a group would break away, forming such new bands as the Many Fat Horses, the All Tall People, and the Knife Owners. On the other hand, the Bear people lost its leading men in a battle in 1872, and its survivors went away to join other bands" (1986, p. 410). Ewers (1946), in his discussion on the Small Robes band, gives a good example of its changing history. He concludes it was at one time a major division of the Blackfoot tribes and that the last surviving families were integrated into other South Peigan bands by 1944.

6 Wissler (1911) mentions twenty band names in his field notes on the South Peigan; two (Seldom Lonesome and No Parfleches) are the same as those mentioned by Grinnell (1962). This suggests that members of these bands separated but kept their old band names. The nineteen band names mentioned by Uhlenbeck (1911) and

the eight on Morgan's list (1964) of the South Peigan, collected in 1862, do not include the same names as Grinnell.

7   For example, Hanks and Hanks (1950) report that eleven bands existed in 1897 for the Blood, but, in 1939, Goldfrank's (1943) informants mention eight existing band names.

8   How the elaborate system of Blood chieftainship changed in a very short period of time is shown by Hanks and Hanks (1950), who mention that "twenty years after treaty, in 1897, there were eleven bands and fourteen chiefs of whom three were elected, six appointed by the agent, and five who had achieved rank in a classical manner." (p. 126)

9   In 1893, Wilson (Godsell 1958) described the social structure of the Blood tribe, where boys of fourteen to twenty years entered the Mosquitos as their first society and then moved on to other society groups. These were, in later years, the Doves (or Pigeons), the Kit Foxes (who amalgamated at a later time with the Horns), the Horns, the Crow Carriers, the Braves, the All Crazy Dogs, and the Catchers. He suggests that the Bulls were the earliest society, but they became obsolete, and members went to the Horns. Fifty years later, Hanks and Hanks (1950) observed that youngest members joined the Bees and finished with the Horns as the highest rank. Most of the old society structures ceased to function, and, after the 1920s, the Prairie Chicken and Crazy Dogs stopped participating in dances. The Horn society eventually included the Kit Foxes, an amalgamation which led to an adaptation of certain aspects of the Sun Dance and the Tobacco Dance. The Buffalo Women or Old Women's society still exists.

10 For example, if an individual defied the Brave Dogs' authority and hunted alone, they would take his horses and weapons. If a man scared away the buffalo, they destroyed his saddle, tipi, and clothes and whipped him. If the Brave Dogs gave an order not to pick berries and a woman disobeyed, they spilled everything that was gathered. If a husband and wife fought and disturbed other people, the Brave Dogs cut their lodges, saddles, and parfleches to pieces. (Parfleches are containers made from buffalo hide and are used to transport goods.)

11 Doty (1966) mentions how, in the early fall of 1855, he met chiefs of several Blackfoot tribes and Bull Head from the North Peigan with his followers in seventy lodges. Doty identifies Bull Head as a band chief. Haydon (1971) mentions Bull Head as the chief of the Undried Meat in Parfleche band. Bull Head met Col. Macleod in 1874 and allowed the NWMP to build a fort on traditional Peigan land, which suggests he was at that time head chief. In 1870, Sees Before and North Axe are mentioned by other authors as leaders of the North Peigan. On the other hand, Sitting on an Eagle Tail and his son North Axe are identified as head chiefs following Bull Head. Other North Peigan leaders who signed Treaty 7 were Many Swans, Morning Plume, and Crow Eagle. MacLean (1893) mentions that Jerry Potts was at one time the war chief of the North Peigan. Ewers' (1947) informant Weasel Tail, a South Peigan, identifies Iron Shirt as chief of the Lone Fighter band. He was originally a Blood but came to live with the North Peigan and later returned to his tribal group.

12 The grandparents were the indulgers of their grandchildren and taught tribal myths and history. It was not unusual for a grandparent to raise one of his or her grandchildren – a custom that is still common today.

13 Women were often married to much older men, and, up to the turn of the century, second or third wives in polygynous marriages were common. All women were expected to behave in a certain manner and be faithful to their husbands and industrious in all their activities. George First Rider (1968) talks about the control and power the husbands had over their wives; "If the girl gets dishonest and her husband catches her in the act she reaches death, her husband will kill her. If her husband doesn't kill her, her brother will kill because they'll be ashamed of her. If her brothers doesn't kill her, her husband will cut off her nose, he will make her eat her own excrement and he will make her drink her urine" (p. 4). Women who did not behave and listen to their husbands had their ears cut off. Sometimes, men were treated

similarly to women for the same offence: "[When a man gets] caught he will be tied to poles with his hands and legs tied apart, he is stripped naked there is nothing on him, his face will be painted with excrement ... the men fart ashes on his face and the ashes will spray on his face, none of his relatives will go up to him because his relatives are ashamed of him, when they are turned loose they go away some never come back they die out in the wilderness because they were embarrassed that is how the first people operate" (First Rider, 1968, pp. 4-5). Duvall (1910) in a letter to Wissler describes similar customs; "When a man finds fault with his wife he simply drives her from his home, sending her back to her people. Once a man found out that his wife was holding company with another man, or had a lover, now this made the husband angry and instead of trying to kill the women, as men usually do, he took his wife and lead [sic] her out by the hand and told her that he was going to make her marry this man, who was her lover. But it happened that the woman's brother heard of this and went over and killed their sister" (pp. 1-2). However, men were treated generally less harshly than women, and disputes over a woman could be settled by the lover giving a horse and other presents to the former husband.

14 Most descriptions and social analyses of Peigan/ Blackfoot culture have been reported by male white observers who, because of their biases, did not understand, see, or have access to a woman's ceremonial roles and sacred status (Kehoe 1976).

15 Again, there were some exceptions. Women from wealthy families who were also in the position to take care of sacred objects according to cultural expectations were sometimes re-married or divorced.

Chapter 4

1 For more detailed information on traditional Peigan/Blackfoot culture, see McClintock (1948, 1968) and Wissler (1911, 1912).

2 As important as the physical manifestation, the Blackfoot worldview attributes an abstract component to each living entity and object, known as "shadow." For this reason, in Blackfoot culture, any manifestation can be explained by being part of the shadow or physical world or both. But moments in time and space when both of these worlds are brought together are regarded as extremely powerful and sacred. Traditional ceremonies are regarded as such occasions and thus have high potential for such benefits as healing or resolving inner or social conflicts for the Peigan community and individuals who ask for help and support.

3 Detailed information on the concept of transfer rites will be discussed in Chapter 5.

4 The Blackfoot Sun Dance ceremony is different from sun dances in other tribes. Based on various cultural adaptations, the presently practised Sun Dance consists of several different sequences, which, at one time, might not have been celebrated together in this form. The first part involves the setting up of camp. The Holy Woman and her companion and supporters then retreat into the Holy Tipi, where she remains secluded for four days. This part of the *Okan* ceremony ends with the cutting and distribution of the tongues, the erection of the centre pole in the middle of the camp, and the blessing and face painting of the people. The second part of the Sun Dance has to do with the dancing of weathermen and members of other societies and with body piercing.

5 McClintock and others comment on the importance of the Holy Woman's fidelity to her husband, and this aspect of the woman's character is re-enacted symbolically in the ceremony. "Their most important ceremonial, the Sundance, began with the vow of a virtuous woman, made for the recovery of the sick. If the patient died, or if disaster came during the ceremonial, as in the case of Good Hunter, the sacred woman killed by lightning, the woman who made the vow was suspected of unchastity. Consequently an unchaste woman would have a superstitious dread of making a vow, or of assuming the part of a sacred woman in a ceremonial. Sickness and death were believed to be the penalties for false vows, visited either upon the woman herself, or upon her relatives" (McClintock 1968, pp. 184–85). This attitude towards women's chastity

was observed by Maximilian zu Wied (1905) and Wilson (1909). "During the time that Scarface was at the Sun's lodge he had been receiving instructions on many religious ceremonials, the most important of which was the *Okan* 'the Sun Dance'. The Sun had said to him, "let no foolish immoral woman make Okan, I will not pay any attention to her prayers. I will only hear the prayers of the wise virtuous women" (Wilson 1909, p. 9).

6 See the detailed account of the origin myth in Appendix C.

7 See Appendix D on Wissler and Duvall's account of the origin of the Sun Dance bundle, recorded as "The Elk Woman."

8 "As previously stated, the natoas ritual in the sun dance has for its mythical basis the Elk-woman and the Woman-who-married-a-star, though Scar-face, Cuts-wood, Otter-woman, and Scabby-round-robe are said to have had minor contributions ... the Woman-who-married-a-star is credited with bringing down the digging-stick and the turnip, together with the songs pertaining thereto, also a wreath of juniper formerly worn in place of the natoas and the eagle feather worn by the man" (Wissler 1918, p. 241).

9 "While the elk-woman is recognized everywhere as the originator of the natoas, it will be noted that the Woman-who-married-a-star is also credited with having contributed the digging stick, the plumes, or leaves of the turnip. The latter seems to have given the name, natoas. In some versions Scar-face is regarded as the child of the woman and also an originator of the bundle. Scabby-round-robe is said to have added the arrow point and the beaverman the tobacco seed, or dwarfs, in the doll's head" (Wissler 1912, p. 215).

10 The Blackfoot had good reason not to disturb the buffalo during that time of the year. In July and August, the buffalo were in their rutting season, and bulls were very aggressive, fighting with each other to gain access to cows. Blackfoot people did not want to endanger their hunters, who might get attacked by bulls, and also did not want to disturb the breeding cycle of the animals.

11 The Holy Woman goes into seclusion for four days while she fasts, not moving and not speaking, but concentrating on prayer.

12 There could have been several *Natoas* in a tribal group that came together, but not all of them were necessarily "activated" at the same time. Once a vow is made with a specific *Natoas*, it needs a separate lodge. However, the *Natoas* that are not activated can, with their present caretakers, support the *Natoas* that is opened in a ceremony.

13 "They taught [Akaiyan] the names of the herbs and roots, which we still use for the curing of the people. They showed him also the different paints, and explained their use, saying, 'If you should use these, they will bring to your people good luck and will ward off sickness and death.' They gave him the seeds of the tobacco (origin of tobacco), and taught him how they should be planted with songs and prayers. They made scratches with their claws on the smooth walls of the lodge to mark the days, and when the days completed a moon, they marked the moon with sticks" (McClintock 1968, p. 108).

14 Some of the most important songs are about the buffalo and other animals that are known to have excellent hunting skills, like weasel or lynx. In the 1965 transfer ceremony of the Calling Last Beaver bundle, the new owner had a lynx tail attached to his hair (McCorquodale 1965).

15 It is interesting to note that, although this is a story related to the South Peigan, the woman seems to belong to the Crow, one of the Blackfoot peoples' foremost enemies. "Now when this woman returned to her people, she started the Crow-water medicine. She is still living among the Crows and the first beaver-skin that came into her hands she kept for medicine" (Wissler and Duvall 1995, p. 78).

16 "In the old days when they were travelling around, and the water is too deep, they'll light up their pipe and hold it in the water and the water goes down. It helped them to survive, almost on an everyday occurrence" (Crowshoe 1997a).

17 Reg Crowshoe remembers the existence of four Beaver bundles alone on the Peigan reserve in Alberta. Hugh Dempsey (no date) reports on a Beaver bundle owned by Charlie Crow Eagle. This bundle previously belonged to Eagle Ribs from Siksika and was at one point given to a North Peigan. The last time it was opened was in 1954, when it was owned by Jim Crow Flag.

Dempsey notes that no one from the North Peigan knew the complete ceremony and songs at the time of Dempsey's visit.

18 Common to all Medicine Pipe bundles is this connection to Thunder, who instructed the first owner in a dream or vision. A vision is usually conceived when a man or a woman goes into seclusion in a remote place and fasts without food or drink for four days. These vision quest sites are primarily located in mountainous areas or on top of hills that overlook and are often in line with specific sites in the Blackfoot heartland. However, a person can also receive instructions in a dream, particularly if dreamt in a painted tipi or in a special location. All forms of vision go through a specific process of verification and interpretation (see Chapter 5 on transfer rites).

19 This pipe is shown in Wied (1976, p. 108) and was likely painted in August or September of 1833. Unfortunately, there is no information on this pipe (for example, its owner or its name). There is a painting of a Blackfoot man with a pipe stem in Catlin (1973), and Paul Kane's painting of a Cree Medicine Pipe bundle is reproduced in his *Wanderings of an Artist* (1968).

20 See Appendix E on the origin myth of the Long Time Pipe by Brings-Down-the-Sun, as told to McClintock (1968).

21 See Appendix F on the accounts collected by Wissler and Duvall (1995).

22 "The pipe is what ties you to Creator. But if you're going to smoke with the Thunder, you better have a real good reason.... If you smoke the pipe and you don't do it with clear intention, you are taking a big risk. You are going to be punished and could be banished from the community. But if you are telling the truth, you are going to get a lot of respect" (Crowshoe 1997b).

23 "The Medicine Pipe was handed down by the thunder, this explains the drumming. The thunder takes nobody for a relative and will electrocute anybody, but he will not molest a woman. The people of the past were afraid of Thunder. When they saw a person's hair stand up they went for safety. A person like this will have blood on him, that's why they are afraid of blood and red cloths cannot be out in the open when it rains" (First Rider 1974).

24 It was the Long Time Pipe that was originally transported on a dog travois and was in the lead when the camp was moved. But once the horse became part of Blackfoot culture, the Riders Pipe was built and took the lead. Another indicator of the older age of the Long Time Pipe shows in the pipe stems and whistles of the respective bundles. The Riders Pipe bundle has rifle barrels for whistles, and pipe stems are often made from metal. In the Long Time Pipe bundles, the materials are wood.

25 "When the first owner of the Catchers Society pipe bundle dreamed about it, the Blackfeet camp was situated about five miles above the site of the present town of Mcleod [Fort Macleod], Alberta, and along Oldman River, at a place called Where They Paint the Raven Lodge. Near this camp was a buffalo fall, called piskun, at the foot of which the chief of the camp had a corral built. He was to direct the ceremony of calling the buffalo over the fall, being the buffalo caller himself. This man dreamed that a little boy came and invited him to his father's lodge. When he went there, he found that the lodge in reality was the piskun. As he entered, he was invited to sit in the rear of the lodge. Many buffalo-people were assembled, and he was informed that they formed the Catchers Society. Each member carried a warclub, at the end of each of which was tied a buffalo-hoof. The leader invited the chief to look up at the top of the lodge, where he saw two pipes hanging; these, he was told, belonged to the leaders of the society. On the first night he was not permitted to witness the entire ceremony; but during the next night he again dreamed that the boy invited him to go to his father's lodge, and this time the pipes were unwrapped and the transfer ceremony was performed. Four times he thus dreamed, and on each occasion was taught the ceremony and the songs. The buffalo-stones are placed in the pipe bundle because the first owner was a caller of buffalo; and for the same reason a buffalo tail is fastened to the pipe" (Wildschut 1912, pp. 423–25).

26 The Black Wrapped pipe was started by Northern Chief, who received it in a dream. It was only to belong to brave, young, and unmarried warriors. It gave success in war and was used

in the capture of enemy horses, and was therefore taken on the warpath. It was said that, if the warriors were surrounded by the enemy, the pipe would save them by making the weather change. It could produce a snowstorm in the wintertime and a cloudburst of rain in the summer; thus, they could escape (Wildschut 1912).

27 "This consists of a rawhide necklace decorated with eight large blue beads and a tubular shell. Hanging from the necklace are two strands of human hair wrapped with yellow and red por-cupine quills. A small bag of red ochre accompanies the necklace. The necklace was given to Mrs. McMaster (*nee* Hazel Black) about 20 years ago when she was a young girl. It was given by a Blackfoot named Maguire whom they called Motokaneepo or Wet Head. He painted the girl and told her she could wear this at any ceremony, particularly at the Sun Dance" (Dempsey 1963).

28 Versions of this story are related in Wissler (1912), Michelson (1916), and Grinnell (1892).

29 It was purchased from Jack Black Horse, a Blackfoot, who inherited the bundle from his mother, but who did not use it, as he "did not have the power that went with it. His mother received this power in a dream" (Dempsey 1963).

30 Duvall wrote to Wissler in 1910 that there were men and women who practised their medicine to prevent women from having children and mentions Old Elk Horn and Jappy as two medicine men with such powers. Virginia Red Crow from Gleichen talks about the Birth Control bundle, which she received from Mrs. Boy Chief, who used her power to control fertility and protect women from conception. (Red Crow 1966).

31 More information on Horse Medicine bundles is found in Ewers (1955) and Wissler (1912).

Chapter 5

1 This would very likely be based on a gender-spe-cific interpretation: men would have to be known for their leadership skills and successes in warfare; women would have to be good role models as homemakers and be faithful to their husbands. It is of special interest to note that two of the Blackfoot cultural heroes, Scarface and Scabby-Round-Robe, do not meet these expectations, but rather were young men who had to go out to prove themselves and were highly rewarded for their courage by receiving sacred bundles through Creator/Sun.

2 "Like other rites this one [weather dancer] was bought and sold, but it was usual to continue in ownership of many years. Anyone could make a vow to dance with the weather dancer and join him in his ceremonies, but such vows were usually made by former owners of the rite. When one makes a vow to purchase the rite, its owner must sell, however reluctant he may be. The transfer must be in the sun dance" (Wissler 1918, p. 260).

3 In fact, the custom of stealing or "capturing" a Medicine Pipe bundle is reflected in the names of many of the Thunder Medicine Pipe bundles; Gros Ventre Pipe, Chippewa Pipe, and so on. There is also the story of how Bird Rattler was able to recapture a Thunder Medicine Pipe that belonged to Big Elk from the Crow which belonged to Big Elk (Schultz 1936) (see Appendix G). However, sometimes medicine pipes were also captured from among the same tribal group. George First Rider (1969) tells the original story of that development.

4 In Western law, copyright is regarded as an individual possession, but, in Blackfoot culture, nothing can be owned individually because everything is "owned" by Creator. A transfer rite gives certain individuals the right to utilize sacred objects and their power in culturally appropriate ways.

5 Horses were adapted to bundles between 1730 and 1800 and were called Riders Medicine Pipe bundles. The old bundles still have parts of dogs (dog tails and hides) and there are dog songs. But many important physical parts of the bundles started to relate to horses. The abstract existence stayed in the songs and the dances. This is reflected in the taboos; for example, bundle owners do not allow dogs inside the house. But many physical components moved on.

6 Appendix H shows how the Small Thunder Medicine Pipe was transferred from its original owner to the present-day owners, Joe and Josephine Crowshoe, in a series of transfer ceremonies.

7 "Cultural confusion comes in when someone comes to a person who has not been given a

transfer ritual and that person paints faces and blesses people. They have not gone through the public acknowledgement of their status; they just go ahead, and they chance their conscience with Creator. But if a person has gone through a transfer ritual they know the rules and regulations and have respect and they would not risk this" (Crowshoe 1996).

8 A public song doesn't have copyright. One can give recognition of the ownership of a song but that recognition is not sacred, which means it has not gone through a transfer rite and is therefore not restricted. Through a transfer rite, a person claims the physical and also the abstract component of a sacred object. If this is done without understanding the power of the process, it is believed that a person will suffer for abusing this principle.

9 "When one asks for help, the person who has gone through the transfer rites should be able to say what they are going to use to help the sick person. It is his responsibility to mention his qualifications. In this case, the protocol would be to ask someone for a sweat and that person would tell you which one they are using based on the transfer ceremony they have gone through. That's why it has to be known publicly and there is a public responsibility. It is his responsibility to say if he can help you or not and perhaps refer you to someone else. This is one of the rules the transfer rituals come with. If I am not doing this publicly my peers can come down on me" (Crowshoe 1996).

Chapter 6

1 These are the roles of the "grandparents," as explained in Chapter 5 on transfer rites.

2 The kind of herbal incense used depended on the kind of bundle present. Nowadays, sweetgrass is used more commonly, especially for personal smudging.

3 Through our research, we observed that the physical handling of the bundle represented Creator's mandate to be held on the women's side. Transferred rites talk about the woman, and the direction given in the songs reinforces the woman's abstract role. The man's mandate is physical, and the songs say that he sits holy. At the same time, he is responsible for leading the process to gather consensus.

4 It is the ceremonialists' role to elicit every participant's opinion on the topic of discussion.

5 This is manifested in the men's and women's equal participation in the process, in how physical presence and abstract thought need to be part of the model, and how material (financial) and personnel contributions need to be incorporated.

6 For example, if a certain plant was in one of the bundles, the physical representation of this plant along with what would be attached to this plant, the songs, and the prayers would entail information on the use, the occurrence, and the spirit of this plant.

Chapter 7

1 In this text, the terms "illness" and "sickness" are used synonymously and describe an individual's experience of pain, stress, and affliction. Illnesses are therefore subjective and defined by an individual's complaints. Diseases are caused by organisms that are introduced to the human body and do not always lead to illness. Environmental factors like poor nutrition, an immune system weakened by other infections, and stressful events affect the body's capability to fight the spread of disease. (Chapter 2 shows how newly introduced viruses like smallpox and measles affected the Peigan.) Disease presents itself not always through physical signs, and, if so, not always in the same way or pattern. Western models of medicine deal with the prevention of disease by boosting the immune system against potential infections and intervening by: (a) introducing other organisms to the human body that fight or suppress an infection, or (b) removing an organism through surgery. The emphasis on pathology within this biomedical health model is, in many ways, in opposition to traditional Blackfoot concepts of curing.

2 These individuals were primarily not medical practitioners but were still likely influenced by their cultural biases and education in relation to health matters.

3 Jack Crow, a seventy-two-year-old North Peigan, speaks on the use of Indian medicine: "Silver root is used on swelling, it is found in the sand hills, dry taste roots are used commonly, wild rose roots are also used 'Soo-yes-sti', or flat lying plants for colds, yellow root, a bitter root grow in swamps, and are used for swelling, bruises and sprains, milk root is known to ease swelling pain, This is found in low lying valleys" (Crow 1973, p. 2).

4 Goldfrank, who collected data on the Blood reserve reports that "both men and women may have medicine for childbirth. Both may have strong power, although some have stronger power than others. Usually we call in a doctor with mild power first. It is cheaper. Only the women doctors give practical help to the woman. The men doctors brew tea and paint the woman's face. This is done when the woman is having a hard time. Then a man with more power will be called in…. One of the midwives cut the cord. A special dressing was put on the cord end and the navel was bound up. The dressing was kept on until the cord broke off. The baby took about twenty-four hours to come. It was a girl." (Goldfrank 1951, p. 87). Other accounts come from Margaret Melting Tallow (1966) and Annie Buffalo (1973), who describe the help of older women during childbirth. They also relate their knowledge to contraceptive methods and fertility charms (Red Crow 1966).

5 Sometimes, these practitioners were also called "shamans" (Brasser 1974, Pringle 1996). However, this term is usually attributed to individuals who go into an altered state, induced either by drugs or by other mechanisms, to diagnose or treat (Chagnon 1977, on Yanomamo; Oppitz 1981, and Watters 1975, on Kham Magar). To use this term to describe the role of the traditional Blackfoot medicine man is therefore misleading. However, a common denominator is their calling to become medical practitioners through a vision that they either sought out actively or that came to them in a dream. (See Wissler's [1912] publication on the experiences of seven Blackfeet medicine men.)

6 "Several hundred spectators, including Indians and traders, were assembled around the dying man, when it was announced that the 'medicine-man' was coming; we were required to 'form a ring,' leaving a space of some thirty or forty feet in diameter around the dying man, in which the doctor could perform his wonderful operations; and a space was also opened to allow him free room to pass through the crowd without touching any one. This being done, in a few moments his arrival was announced by the death-like 'hush – sh –', through the crowd; and nothing was to be heard, save the light and casual tinkling of the rattles upon his dress, which was scarcely perceptible to the ear, as he cautiously and slowly moved through the avenue left for him; which at length brought him into the ring, in view of the pitiable object over whom his mysteries were to be performed….

His entree and his garb were somewhat thus: – he approached the ring with his body in a crouching position, with a slow and tilting step – his body and head were entirely covered with the skin of a yellow bear, the head of which (his own head being inside of it) served as a mask; the huge claws of which also were dangling on his wrists and ankles; in one hand he shook a frightful rattle, and in the other brandished his medicine-spear or magic wand; to the rattling din and discord of all of which, he added the wild and startling jumps and yelps of the Indian, and the horrid and appalling grunts, and snarls, and growls of the grizzly bear, in ejaculatory and guttural incantations to the Good and Bad Spirits, in behalf of his patient; who was rolling and groaning the agonies of death, whilst he was dancing around him, jumping over him, and pawing him about, and rolling him in every direction.

In this wise, this strange operation proceeded for half and hour, to the surprise of a numerous and death-like silent audience, until the man died; and the medicine-man danced off to his quarters, and packed up, and tied and secured from the sight of the world, his mystery dress and equipments" (Catlin 1973, pp. 39–40).

7 "A number of wounded men, women, and children, were laid or placed against the walls; others, in their deplorable condition, were pulled about by their relations, amid tears and lamentations.

The White Buffalo, whom I have often mentioned, and who had received a wound at the back of his head, was carried about, in this manner, amid singing, howling and crying: they rattled the *schischikue* in his ears, that the evil spirit might not overcome him, and gave him brandy to drink. He himself, though stupefied and intoxicated, sung without intermission, and would not give himself up to the evil spirit ... instead of suffering the wounded, who were exhausted by the loss of blood, to take rest, their relations continually pulled them about, sounded large bells, rattled their medicine or amulets, among which were the bears' paws, which the White Buffalo wore on his breast" (Maximilian zu Wied 1905, p. 148).

8 But there seem to have also been areas of specialization for the curing of specific body parts and health problems, for instance, the head, the lungs, and intestinal/digestive troubles (George First Rider, Jan. 4, no date).

9 "The Indian Medicine Man played a prominent part among these people in the early years. He was supposed to cure all ailments from headaches to tuberculosis, but he never attempted any surgery. His treatments were varied, according to the trouble. If it were the last stages of tuberculosis, he would lean over the patient's body with a rattle made of the dried bladder of an animal in which were placed several small stones. This was tied to a wooden handle about six inches long. This rattle would be shaken over the patient's body for hours, the idea being to keep away the evil spirits. Sometimes the Medicine Man would put his mouth on the patient's chest to suck away the poison, as he called it. While this performance was going on, the small room was usually filled with relations and friends of the sick person, many of them smoking. Of course there were other methods of treatment, some of which were effective. They used wild strawberry for dysentery and other herbs to apply to the forehead when headache was the trouble" (Graham 1991, p. 44).

10 It could have been that Denny did not see a white mouse but rather a white weasel, which was used for curing in the following way: "The weasel is about two hundred years old. It was passed down by the owner Yellow Comes Over Hill.

When different tribes were at war, he was well known for healing the wounded with this weasel. He performed his healing by covering the weasel with a cloth. Once covered the weasel would move and run to the wound of a man. It would move about the wound leaving it without a single trace of the wound except for a yellow stain as if it was painted. Then it would run back to where it was covered, drop down and is just a stuffed weasel again" (Bull Bear 1965).

11 "An old man named Calf Shirt, snake charmer, showed off a tame rattlesnake that he always carries on his person. Another, a relative of Red Crow named Kakko-Stamik, specializes in handling without fear these kinds of deadly snakes. He either has a medicine or a gift to instantly heal the bite of these terrible reptiles ... that is what these Indians claim, at last" (Doucet, no date, p. 14).

12 "My father's mother's mother had a skunk pelt which she used for curing. The skunk pelt comes alive if she used all her power. Even if the patient is very sick, if he has pneumonia or some other severe illness. If the pelt comes alive that means she is going to have success in curing the patient and if the skunk pelt should not come alive it is a very bad omen, the patient will not recover. The skunk pelt would jump up and start running and my grandmother would utter a sound of praise and satisfaction. This skunk pelt was given to me as a charm, it's just a head piece. They say that I was always sick when I was a child. My grandmother said that I would grow up; "He will live." The charm was tied on me and my face was painted and I grew up. I used to have braids and I tied the skunk pelt to my braids, the skunk is complete" (Black Plume 1967).

13 "The object is known in Blackfoot as *Ekuk-ksis-tukee*, or Little Beaver. It was owned by Kyso-tamiso, or Came from Above. He was a great-uncle of Amos Leather. This man was a great medicine man and doctor of the Blackfoot Indians and died shortly after the Blackfoot Treaty was signed. The Little Beaver was used in curing people who were ill. A sick person or member of the family would call on Came from Above and he would come to the bedside of the afflicted Indian. A special song which goes with

the Little Beaver was sung and the patient was painted with a special dark red paint which went with the skin. This paint was rubbed on the forehead in an upward motion and on the backs of each of the hands. The Little Beaver was then hung around the neck of the patient and placed under their left armpit. There it remained until the patient was cured. For his services Came from Above would be paid two or three horses or a mare and its colts. He was paid regardless of whether the person survived. Came from Above was the only person who had the power to use the Little Beaver for curative purposes. After his death it passed down through various members of the family and was then given to Amos Leather's daughter by a female relative. It might be mentioned that there were three brothers in the family, all of whom were medicine men. These were Came from Above, Kyso-tamiso; Sepisto-kossi, or Owl Child; Mee-now-yee or Berry Eater. The latter was Amos' grand-father" (Dempsey 1961).

14 "This feather is put in water, and this one you put a little bit out of this and chew it until it is fine. This one will be chewed, the patient will be lying on the bed, and where the pain is, in the stomach or on the chest or in the head. This one will be chewn. This fungus will be scraped fine somewhat like flour. Then a hot charcoal will be put in to a pan and the scrapings from the fungus will be put over the hot charcoal and you will put your hand over the smoke. Now if this root has been chewn and then you will blow it on where the pain is and then you will put your hand on the patient where the pain is with the bone blower tube. Now this paint. The patient will be painted on the forehead on both cheeks and on the chin. After the treatment the patient will get up. Now this shell. You will chew some of this root, the shell will be heated red hot and what is chewn from the root will be put into the shell and this will be laid on where the pain is with the chewn root against the skin and the shell on top and it will be tied on the patient. It will be painful but he will not get burned. This feather is for washing off the spot where the treatment is going to be, hands are not used. Yes, it's an owl's feather. A sick person is so very tender he doesn't want to be hurt. That is why this feather is used.

After a while the medicine will bother him and it will be taken off. That's all" (Black 1967).

15 Several authors report that as a sign of mourning, people would amputate the last part of their little finger and that they used sharp flints for these amputations before the usage of knives. "I have told you how men are called upon to cut off pieces of skin and how certain old women were selected to amputate fingers. You should also know that in olden times there were some women and men who might be called upon to cut open dead persons for various reasons. Sometimes they did this on their own account in order to get information as to the cause of death" (Wissler 1918, p. 267). Traditionally, flints and eagle claws were and are used to cut the muscles during the torture part of the *Okan*.

16 "I might feel your chest and find your sickness. Then I will get a flint crystal knife and pull up the skin over sick region and puncture it. It is a little puncture. Then I will suck out the blood that flows and spit it away. Now the sickness will come out in the blood and the patient will heal. Then I will take the roots that I was given in my dream and that I keep in my little bags, and chew them up. The wounds are spit upon with that." (First Rider, no date).

17 See Appendix I on how the curative skill of bone setting was practised and transferred from father to son.

18 These types of bundles are mentioned in Chapter 4 and categorized as personal bundles. In this case, it is again the weasel spirit's power that is used for the curing procedure (see Appendix I).

19 "This outfit is called '*eetah-sikin-akyop*', or 'doctor's kit'. It was used by Jack's mother, Antelope Woman, the wife of Black Horse. Jack inherited this, but did not use it because he did not have the power that went with it. His mother received this power in a dream. The kit was used for a variety of ailments, but was most commonly used in the treatment of pneumonia. Jack had participated in the ceremonies, as a drummer, and was able to describe the procedure. His mother would begin by heating a single large stone. While Jack drummed and sang, she would take the hair from the kit and put it into her mouth. She would take the long bone tube and blow

upon the sore or infected area. This would cause a deep, penetrating heat. A vessel was placed upon the hot stone and some water was heated. When hot, some of the root in the kit was mixed with tobacco and added to the water. The root is called *mamyokuki* or 'fish back'. His mother took the feather and dipped into the contents of the vessel. She (patted) the moisture on to the infected area in this manner. After treating the patient in this manner, she would take the tiny stone and place it on the infected area. If it stood up, it indicated that the patient was recovering; if it fell over, the medication was not taking effect. Jack stated that one of Mrs. Gunny Crow's children was one of the last people that his mother cured with this outfit. The bone tube, which is tapered at both ends, was used to suck the pain or evil from a sick person during treatment. Human hair, usually from the patient, was brushed over the infected area, and a tube placed against the spot. By sucking, the doctor could draw out the cause of illness. This tube appears to be a hair bone which was handled by traders and used for making breast ornaments" (Dempsey 1963).

20 Another example of how a medicine man was able to predict future events is recorded by Fidler (1991), who met the Peigan in January 1793 and tells about a medicine man who is asked to foresee if some young men who went on the warpath are coming back. This is done in a shaking tent ceremony.

21 As men and women play leading roles as ceremonialists in Blackfoot culture, traditional medical practitioners can be men or women. However, women were primarily active in childbirth and men in surgery, especially around ceremonial piercing. Maximilian zu Wied (1905) observes how "Otsequa-Stomik, an old man of our acquaintance, was wounded in the knee by a ball, which a woman cut out with a penknife, during which operation he did not betray the least symptoms of pain" (p. 148).

22 "The Chief says that in the old days the Blackfoots observed a very rigid course of personal hygiene including, for all men and boys, a daily morning bath, summer or winter, in cold water. This cold plunge, which often required that a hole be chopped in the ice, was believed by the Blackfoots to toughen them against extremely cold weather and to build their resistance to various winter ailments. The Chief says that it worked, too, and that when the Blackfoots were allowed to exist in their traditional manner, living in teepees which were lined, and floored with furs, and snug as a jug, and eating their customary diet of meat supplemented with a variety of esculent wild fruits, berries, roots and tubers, such disorders as pneumonia and the common cold were almost unheard of. But then came the White Man, awooing with his plea of 'Let me take all this away from you'. And that is exactly what he did. The Chief remembers the old days very well, and his voice took on an understandably bitter edge as he explained the extent to which the White Man's senseless slaughter of the buffalo destroyed the Blackfoot way of life. Other game could not even begin to meet the food needs of the Plains Tribes. With the buffalo gone the Indians were forced to accept the refined foods of the White Man; with no buffalo hides with which to build lodges, the Indians were forced to live in smoky, unventilated wooden shacks. Consequently, the Indians began to suffer terribly from such diseases as pneumonia, appendicitis, tuberculosis, and trachoma. Additional gifts from the Whites in the form of alcohol and smallpox conspired with other catastrophes to reduce the Blackfoots, once the most populous and powerful of all Plains Tribes and believed by some historians to have numbered at one time over forty thousand, to fewer than five thousand souls. The Indian was robbed of the natural resources and the *lebensraum* that were his rightful heritage, and then he was denied the wherewithal and the knowledge, and the motivation, to live any other kind of life" (Lancaster 1966, p. 118).

23 Two of his more regular patients were Crowfoot and one of his sons, whom he treated for headaches and eye problems. Other health problems were injuries, inflammation of the lungs, hemorrhaging, and an epidemic of influenza.

24 In 1877, Nevitt treats Crowfoot in his camp and observes that "he is suffering considerably from sciatica; found the drums going and a medicine woman burning little holes in his leg along the course of the pain" (p. 13). "I found Brown's

Indian wife suffering from a severe attack of this epidemic Influenza.... Her nose was bleeding copiously. She had Indian doctors attending to her and they effected no relief" (Nevitt 1974, p. 90).

25 "One of the most noticeable conditions of Indian life in those early years and for several years later was their poverty.... Tuberculosis and scrofula were rampant and medical attention was at rare intervals. A medical man visited the reserve once a month and remained for only an hour or so, according to the train service.... an epidemic of measles broke out among the children in our vicinity" (Stocken 1976, pp. 12–13).

26 "There was never real medical service, sometimes a doctor would travel through the reserve. He never told anyone to go to the hospital. He gave castor oil to the children. The Indians called him 'Castor Oil Doctor'. Many times the Indian doctor saved their own people, so most of the Indians used their own doctor's methods. They crushed roots and herb and then heated them in rock and water and benefited from the evaporation of the steam" (Buffalo, no date).

27 "I am able to care for them when their sicknesses are not too serious. Since they have been confined to reserve, however, the health condition of the Blackfoot people, as well as of other Indian people living in similar situations, is deteriorating very rapidly. Accustomed to a nomadic way of living, they are not able to adjust to the inconveniences of a more inactive life. In winter, their lodgings are dirty, too cramped for the number of people, over-heated ... and with inadequate nourishment, besides. All of this becomes a breeding ground for scroful, enteristis, lung and skin infections, and even, in too many cases, the kinds of bad diseases that loose-living white people have given them. Beside this, some unscrupulous companies, or at least their merchants, have been furnishing them with spoiled food supplies" (Doucet, no date, p. 46).

28 "It was operated by two English Nurses who were called Sisters. The doctor from Pincher Creek came once in a while. These Sisters used to teach the Indians how to care for minor sores and cuts and also dispensed drugs. There were beds for people who needed Hospital care, but very few stayed. Drugs dispensed were, castor oil, Epsom salts, Cod Liver Oil, aspirins, vasline and eye medications. Later these Sisters left" (English and Potts 1984).

29 Eddy Yellow Horn mentions that Three Horses went in 1925 to Calgary to meet with the Minister of Indian Affairs (Charlie Stewart) to ask for a new hospital and school, which were built the following year.

30 The federal government maintains the position that First Nations members have no right *per se* to provision of medical services. This opinion is in contradiction to the position taken by First Nations governments. They claim that the signing of the treaties included the right to comprehensive medical care. (See Chapter 2 on the different perspectives between Blackfoot people and the Canadian government pertaining to the treaty promises made.)

Chapter 8

1 Only a minority of residents fully understand the existing health system. They are mostly individuals who have been trained and educated in Western structures of learning, such as colleges, universities, or other organizations.

2 And, as pointed out previously, this model is not limited to the area of health management, but may be applied to all other areas of organizational structuring and may be used in many other Native communities – possibly all groups that had a ceremonial format similar to that of the Blackfoot people.

3 For example, we recommend that the Blackfoot Circle Structure also be used for the health needs assessment of the Peigan community. In this case, some of the supporting positions will be different from the main health service structure model. Various other knowledgeable supporters might be invited to join the group on an occasional basis.

4 Who specifically takes this place depends upon the topic of the meeting. For example, if the topic is more strongly related to traditional issues, Reg Crowshoe would be appropriate in this role, and if it is more health related, Sybille Manneschmidt would be the person to join.

5 Comparably, in court and other legal proceedings, it is the gavel used by the judge that starts the court process.

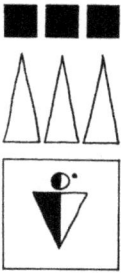

Bibliography

Baur, Susan. 1991. *The Dinosaur Man: Tales of Madness and Enchantment from the Back Ward*. New York: HarperCollins.

Berreman, G. D. 1968. Ethnolography: Method and Product. In *Introduction to Cultural Anthropology*, edited by J. Clifton. Boston: Houghton Mifflin.

Berry, Gerald L. 1953. *The Whoop-Up Trail: (Alberta-Montana Relationships)*. Edmonton: Applied Art Products.

Black, Francis. 1967. Shamanism [Interview].

Black Plume, Bob. 1967. Shamanism [Interview].

Brasser, Ted J. 1974. Wolf Collar: The Shaman as Artist. *ArtsCanada* 30 (5-6).

Brink, Jack. 1992. Blackfoot and Buffalo Jumps. In *Buffalo*, edited by J. E. Foster, D. Harrison and I. S. MacLaren. Edmonton: University of Alberta Press.

Browne, John M. 1866. Indian Medicine. *Atlantic Monthly* 7.

Buffalo, Annie. 1973. Birth Control [Interview].

Bull Bear, David. 1965. Explanation of the Function of the Weasel War Charm [Interview], July 2.

Bullchild, Percy. 1985. *The Sun Came Down*. New York: Harper & Row.

Canada. Department of Indian Affairs. 1880. Annual Report for 1879. Edgar Dewdney to Sir John A. Macdonald.

Catlin, George. 1973. *Letters and Notes on the Manners, Customs, and Condition of the North American Indians: 1832-39*. New York: Dover.

Chagnon, Napoleon A. 1977. *Yanomamö: The Fierce People, Case Studies in Cultural Anthropology*. New York: Holt Rinehart and Winston.

Crow, Jack. 1973. Treaty 7 [Interview], January 1.

Crowshoe, Reg. 1996. Copyright Definitions [Interview], March 11.

———. 1997a. Bundles [Interview].

———. 1997b. Thunder Medicine Pipe and Natoas Bundles [Interview].

———. 1997e. Creation Story [Interview].

Dempsey, Hugh A. 1961. Memo to W. Fleming "Little Beaver Skin".

———. 1962. Blackfoot Medicine Pipe Bundle [Report].

———. 1963. Blacktail Deer Dance Rattle [Observation].

———. 1964. David Thompson under Scrutiny. *Alberta Historical Review* 12 (1).

———. 1965. *A Blackfoot Winter Count, Occasional Paper; no. 1*. Calgary: Glenbow Foundation.

———. 1986. The Blackfoot Indians. In *Native Peoples: The Canadian Experience*, edited by R. B. Morrison and C. R. Wilson. Toronto: McClelland and Stewart.

———. 1988. *Indian Tribes of Alberta*. Calgary: Glenbow Museum.

———. no date. Horse Medicine Bundle [Report].

Denny, Cecil E. Sir. 1944. Blackfoot Magic. *The Beaver*.

———. 1972. *The Law Marches West*. 2 ed. Toronto: Dent.

Doty, J. A. 1966. Visit to the Blackfoot Camps. *Alberta Historical Review* 14 (3).

Doucet. no date. My Journals: Excerpts from Father Doucet's Missionary Journals. Edmonton: Provincial Museum and Archives of Alberta.

Dunn, Jack F. 1994. *The Alberta Field Force of 1885*. Calgary: Jack Dunn.

Duvall, D. C. 1910. Letter to Wissler.

———. 1911. Letter to Wissler.

———. 1936. Anthropological archives. New York: American Museum of Natural History.

English, E., and V. Potts. 1984. Development of Health Services—Peigan Reserve [Report].

Ewers, John Canfield. 1946. Identification and History of Small Robes Band of the Peigan. *Journal of the Washington Academy of Sciences* 36 (12).

———. 1947. Some Winter Sports of Blackfoot Indian Children. *The Masterkey* 47.

———. 1949. The Last Bison Drives of the Blackfoot Indians. *Journal of the Washington Academy of Sciences* 39 (11).

———. 1955. The Horse in Blackfoot Indian Culture. *Bureau of American Ethnology. Bulletin (Washington)* 159.

———. 1962. Mothers of the Mixed Bloods. *El Palicio: A Quarterly Journal of the Museum of New Mexico* 69 (1).

Fidler, Peter. 1991. *Southern Alberta Bicentennial: A Look at Peter Fidler's Journal: Journal of a Journey over Land from Buckingham House to the Rocky Mountains in 1792 & 3*. Edited by B. Haig. 2nd ed. Lethbridge, Alta.: Historical Research Centre.

First Rider, George. 1968. Mourning Rites [Interview].

———. 1969. The Medicine Pipe of the Blood Indians [Interview], April 30.

———. 1974. Medicine Pipe Bundle [Observation], August.

———. no date. Medicinal Practices [Interview], January 4, 19??

Frantz, Donald G., and Norma Jean Russell. 1989. *Blackfoot Dictionary of Stems, Roots, and Affixes*. Toronto: University of Toronto Press.

Fraser, Fran. no date. Tobacco Bundles [Report].

Frisch, R. 1975. Critical Weights: A Critical Body Composition, Menarche, and the Maintenance of Menstrual Cycles. In *Biosocial Interrelations in Population Adaptation*, edited by E. S. Watts, F. E. Johnston and G. W. Lasker. The Hague: Mouton.

Frisch, R. et al. 1974. Menstrual Cycles: Fatness as a Determinant of Minimum Weight for Height Necessary for their Maintenance or Onset. *Science* 185.

Gambler, Joe. 1968. Long Time Pipe [Interview].

Godsell, P. H. 1958. *The R. N. Wilson Papers*. Calgary: Glenbow Museum.

Goldfrank, Esther Schiff. 1943. Administrative Programs and Changes in Blood Society during the Reserve Period. *Applied Anthropology* 2.

———. 1951. Observations on Sexuality among the Blood Indians of Alberta, Canada. *Psychoanalysis and the Social Sciences* 3.

Graham, William M. 1991. *Treaty Days: Reflections of an Indian Commissioner*. Calgary: Glenbow Museum.

Gray, James Henry. 1971. *Red Lights on the Prairies*. Toronto: Macmillan.

Grinnell, George Bird. 1892. Early Blackfoot History. *American Anthropologist* 5.

———. 1962. *Blackfoot Lodge Tales: The Story of a Prairie People*. Lincoln, Neb.: University of Nebraska.

Hale, H. 1885. Report on the Blackfoot Tribes: On the North-Western Tribes and the Dominion of Canada.

Hanks, Lucien Mason, and Jane Hanks. 1950. *Tribe Under Trust: A Study of the Blackfoot Reserve of Alberta*. Toronto: University of Toronto Press.

Haydon, Arthur Lincoln. 1971. *The Riders of the Plains: A Record of the Royal North-West Mounted Police of Canada, 1873-1910*. Edmonton: Hurtig.

Hellson, John C. 1966. Report on the Transferal Ceremony of the Big Corner Post Drum. Edmonton: Provincial Museum and Archives of Alberta.

Hellson, John C., and Morgan Gadd. 1974. *Ethnobotany of the Blackfoot Indians, Canadian Ethnology Service Paper no. 19. Mercury Series*. Ottawa: National Museums of Canada.

Higinbotham, John David. 1978. *When the West Was Young: Historical Reminiscences of the Early Canadian West*. 2nd ed. Lethbridge, Alta.: Herald.

Jenness, Diamond. 1955. *The Indians of Canada.* 3rd ed, *National Museum of Canada. Bulletin 65; Anthropological Series, no. 15.* Ottawa: Cloutier.

de Josselin de Jong, J.P.B. 1914. Blackfoot Texts. *Verhandelingen der Koninklijke Akademie van Wetenschappen te Amsterdam, Afdeelingletterkunde* 14 (4).

Kane, Paul. 1968. *Wanderings of an Artist among the Indians of North America: from Canada to Vancouver's Island and Oregon Through the Hudson's Bay Company's Territory and Back Again.* Edmonton: Hurtig.

Kehoe, Alice B. 1976. Old Women Had Great Power. *Western Canadian Journal of Anthropology* 6 (3).

———. 1993. How the Ancient Peigans Lived. *Research in Economic Anthropology* 14.

Kelsey, Henry. 1929. *The Kelsey Papers.* Edited by A. G. Doughty and C. Martin. Ottawa: F. A. Acland.

Kipp, Jack. 1965. Medicine Pipe Transfer [Observation].

Lancaster, Richard. 1966. *Peigan: A Look from Within at the Life, Times, and Legacy of an American Indian Tribe.* sl.: sn.

Legal, Emile. 1885. 1885 Field Notes on Customs, Legends and Other Stories among the Blackfoot Peoples [Report].

Lewis, Oscar. 1941. Manly-Hearted Women among the North Peigan. *American Anthropologist* 43.

MacGregor, J. G. 1949. *Blankets and Beads: A History of the Saskatchewan River, Peel Bibliography on Microfiche; no. 4163.* Edmonton: Institute of Applied Art.

MacLean, John. 1893. *Social Organization of the Blackfoot Indians.* s.l.: s.n.

Manneschmidt, Sybille M. K. 1994. Wombs and Witches: Important Aspects of Kham Magar Women's Health, Fertility and Reproduction. Ph.D., University of Alberta, Edmonton.

McClintock, Walter. 1935. *The Blackfoot Beaver Bundle, Southwest Museum Leaflets; no. 2–3.* Los Angeles: Southwest Museum.

———. 1948. *Blackfoot Medicine-Pipe Ceremony, Southwest Museum Leaflets; no. 21.* Los Angeles: Southwest Museum.

———. 1968. *The Old North Trail: Or, Life, Legends and Religion of the Blackfeet Indians.* Lincoln, Neb.: University of Nebraska.

———. 1969. *Dances of the Blackfoot Indians, Southwest Museum Leaflets; no. 7.* Los Angeles: Southwest Museum.

McCorquodale, B. A. 1965. Calling Last Beaver Bundle Transfer [Observation].

Melting Tallow, David. 1966. Medicine Pipe Transferal Ceremony of the Blackfoot Proper [Observation], September 25.

———. 1967. Medicine Pipe Bundle Transfer [Observation].

Melting Tallow, Margaret. 1966. Beaver Bundle [Observation].

Michelson, T. 1916. *Notes on the Peigan System of Consanguinity.* Washington: Bureau of American Ethnology.

Middleton, E. D. 1953. History, Evolution and Culture of the Blood Indians. *Lethbridge Herald.*

Morgan, Lewis Henry. 1964. *Ancient Society, John Harvard Library.* Cambridge, Mass.: Belknap Press of Harvard University Press.

Mountain Horse, Mike. 1979. *My People the Bloods.* Calgary: Glenbow-Alberta Institute.

Nevitt, R. B. 1974. *A Winter at Fort Macleod.* Edited by H. A. Dempsey. Calgary: Glenbow-Alberta Institute.

Oppitz, M. 1981. *Schamanen im Blinden Land.* Frankfurt: Syndikat Verlag.

Potyondi, Barry. 1992. *Where the Rivers Meet: A History of the Upper Oldman River Basin to 1939.* Lethbridge, Alta.: Robins Southern Printing.

Pringle, Heather Anne. 1996. *In Search of Ancient North America: An Archaeological Journey to Forgotten Cultures.* New York: John Wiley & Sons.

Raczka, Paul M. 1979. *Winter Count: A History of the Blackfoot People.* Brocket, Alta.: Oldman River Culture Centre.

Ray, Arthur J. 1996. *I Have Lived Here Since the World Began: An Illustrated History of Canada's Native Peoples.* Toronto: Lester Publishing.

Red Crow, Virginia. 1966. Birth Control Bundle [Interview], February 2.

Samek, Hana. 1987. *The Blackfoot Confederacy, 1880-1920: A Comparative Study of Canadian and U.S. Indian Policy.* Albuquerque: University of New Mexico Press.

Schultz, James Willard. 1930. *The Sun God's Children.* Boston: Houghton Mifflin.

———. 1936. Thunder Pipe. *Great Falls Tribune,* March 22.

Smith, Nick. no date. Societies [Interview].

Spry, Irene M. 1963. *The Palliser Expedition: An Account of John Palliser's British North American Expedition, 1857-1860.* Toronto: Macmillan.

Steele, Samuel Benfield. 1915. *Forty Years in Canada: Reminiscences of the Great North-West, with Some Account of his Service in South Africa, By Colonel S.B. Steele... Late of the N.W.M Police.* Edited by M. G. Niblett. London: Herbert Jenkins.

Stocken, H. W. Gibbon. 1976. *Among the Blackfoot and Sarcee.* Calgary: Glenbow Alberta Institute.

Sully, General. 1870. Census of Blackfoot Indians, July 16, 1870 [Report]. Washington: Office of Indian Affairs Records, National Archives.

Taylor, Jack Leonard. 1987. Two Views on the Meaning of Treaties Six and Seven. In *The Spirit of the Alberta Indian Treaties,* edited by R. Price. Edmonton: Pica Pica Press.

Tims, John William. 1889. *Grammar and Dictionary of the Blackfoot Language in the Dominion of Canada, Peel Bibliography on Microfiche; no. 1130.* London: Society for Promoting Christian Knowledge.

Turner, John Peter. 1950. *The North-West Mounted Police, 1873-1893, Peel Bibliography on Microfiche; no. 4226.* Ottawa: King's Printer.

Uhlenbeck, Christianus Cornelius. 1911. *Original Blackfoot Texts from the Southern Peigans Blackfoot Reservation, Teton County, Montana, Akademie van Wetenschappen, Amsterdam. Afdeeling voor de Taal-, Letter-, Geschiedkundige in Wijsgeerige Wetenschappen. Verhandelingen. Nieuwe reeks, deel 12, no. 1.* Amsterdam: J. Müller.

Watters, D. 1975. Siberian Shamanistic Traditions among the Kham Magar of Nepal. *Contributions to Nepalese Studies 2.*

Wied, Maximilian. 1905. *Maximilian, Prince of Wied's Travels in the Interior of North America, 1832-1834.* Vol. 23, *Early Western Travels, 1748-1846.* Cleveland: Arthur H. Clark.

———. 1976. *People of the First Man: Life among the Plains Indians in their Final Days of Glory: The Firsthand Account of Prince Maximilian's Expedition up the Missouri River, 1833-34.* Edited by D. Thomas and K. Ronnefeldt. New York: Dutton.

Wildschut, William. no date. Indian Notes [Report].

Wilson, Robert N. 1909. The Sacrificial Rite of the Blackfoot [Report]: Royal Society of Canada, Sec. 2.

———. 1921. *Our Betrayed Wards: A Story of 'Chicanery, Infidelity and the Prostitution of Trust', Peel Bibliography on Microfiche; no. 2798.* Ottawa: s.n.

Wissler, Clark. 1910. *Material Culture of the Blackfoot Indians.* Vol. 5, pt. 1, *Anthropological Papers of the American Museum of Natural History.* New York: s.n.

———. 1911. *The Social Life of the Blackfoot Indians.* Vol. 7, pt. 1, *Anthropological Papers of the American Museum of Natural History.* sl.: sn.

———. 1912. *Ceremonial Bundles of the Blackfoot Indians.* Vol. 7, pt. 2, *Anthropological Papers of the American Museum of Natural History.* New York: s.n.

———. 1913. *Societies and Dance Associations of the Blackfoot Indians.* Vol. 11, pt. 4, *Anthropological Papers of the American Museum of Natural History.* New York: s.n.

———. 1918. *The Sun Dance of the Blackfoot Indians.* Vol. 16, pt. 3, *Anthropological Papers of the American Museum of Natural History.* New York: s.n.

———. 1941. *North American Indians of the Plains.* 3d ed, *Handbook Series (American Museum of Natural History), no. 1.* New York.

Wissler, Clark, and D. C. Duvall. 1995. *Mythology of the Blackfoot Indians, Sources of American Indian Oral Literature.* Lincoln, Neb.: University of Nebraska Press.

www.ingramcontent.com/pod-product-compliance
Lightning Source LLC
Chambersburg PA
CBHW081403270326
41930CB00015B/3393